Natural BOOK of CURES

BY
TERRY COOKSEY

A Health and Food Guide to Cure and Prevent Most Diseases and Medical Conditions

Ingram Content Group – Lightning Source Edition

COVER ART BY
TERRY COOKSEY

www.AmericanPublishing.us
inquiries@americanpublishing.us

THERE IS A CURE FOR EVERY DISEASE

ISBN-13: 978-1-939147-40-0
ISBN-10:   1-939147-40-9

Natural Healing – BOOK of CURES

A Health and Food Guide to Cure and Prevent

Most Diseases and Medical Conditions

Table of Contents

ISBN-13: 978-1-939147-40-0

ISBN-10: 1-939147-40-9

1 - Introduction – Why this book was written

The information in this book can cure you of every disease you have, naturally, since practically all disease is caused by poisons. The general idea of this book comes from holistic medicine and the natural cures and treatments man used throughout history until about 1939. This was where medicine and health care got derailed down the path of greed and love of money, and your health became more and more irrelevant to this new modern faux medical profession that abandoned all cures and natural medicines starting in 1939.

Their entire scope of methods are all synthetic harmful substitutes for the natural methods and natural medicines man ever knew until 1939. And just about everything left in the medical profession are man-made and synthetic. The drugs doctors prescribe as the foundation of their medical profession are all removed by your body and never become a part of your body. But with natural medicines, herbs, our bodies use the ingredients in those herbs and do become part of our body.

There is no bashing, mis-informing anyone about doctors or intent to incite people to do anything about doctors and their helpless medical profession in this book. Everything I say about doctors are facts we all know are true, but for various irrational reasons, people have different rules for doctors than they do for any other group of people. The fact is that there would be no real use for books about cures IF doctors of today would cure us.

If you're seriously looking for a cure, then this book is about the best information you could have, since doctors pretty much have no cures.

Which would you choose? A cure for pennies a day? Or treatment of your disease for thousands of dollars every year or so? I cured myself of "incurable" bladder stones back in 1996 after having four episodes of bladder stones in the three years prior to curing myself. I also cured myself of twenty years of daily heartburn (acid reflux), headaches 4 or 5 times a week, arthritic swollen joints 4 or 5 days a week and other conditions which I will tell you about later on. Remember, this is just an introduction to give you a good idea and foundation of what this book is about and why you might be interested in reading on.

So who will this book benefit? The easy answer to that is all humans and some pets. But in reality, those who will value this book the most are those who don't like to suffer, don't like paying doctor and hospital bills, those who can't afford health care, those who need information in their pursuit of natural methods and cures and the holistic approach. The holistic approach is that disease and its symptoms are just signs of a whole body problem. So you repair the body naturally, which in turn alleviates the symptoms of diseases.

What I do not find in holistic medicine is talk about avoiding the poisons that saturate our food, drinks and water supplies in America and our hygiene items and over the counter medications like soap, shampoo, toothpaste, deodorant, aspirin, acetaminophen, ibuprofen and naproxen. This is in no way a criticism of holistic medicine. It's merely pointing out **the main focus of this book - teaching people to find the poisons in products you use and avoiding those products, as well as giving you information to find healthier product substitutes, while making sure you learn how to meet the basic needs of your body.**

Although the results of you following the advice, facts and/or opinions stated in this book will sometimes seem like a miracle cure, in all honesty, there are two main facts to remember about your results: 1) Your results will depend on how well you limit or eliminate poisons and 2) How well you adjust your diet and take supplements to correct deficiencies in your diet. It's all up to you to put this information to work in your life and your families' lives. Just as you are stuffing your faces with large amounts of toxic, disease causing poisons, now you can choose to stop stuffing those poisons down your own throats!

And guess what! If you wanna know who is responsible for you being sick, then grab a mirror and take a look! It's YOU! YOU made YOU sick. But the great news is that you can make yourself well and cure yourself; and do so at a tiny fraction of the cost of insurance, doctor bills, hospital bills and the likes. You just need some help getting the right information. And that's where this book will help you in major ways.

A whole lot of people will think this is a DIET book. But if you think about that as you read this book, you will quickly see that this book is about reducing the amounts of poisons in your food, drinks and water supplies you consume that are the CAUSE of at least 80% of all disease.

These poisons saturate everything; even our hygiene items like underarm deodorants, soap, shampoo, makeup and so much more. Your body can only remove a certain amount of these poisons. Most do OK until they get in their late 20's and beyond. As resilient as our bodies are, the huge overload of poisons begin to form diseases in our bodies once we have brought them into an acidic disease state. Once our bodies are acidic by eating and drinking all that sugar, high fructose corn syrup, meat and other animal products, those poisons begin to damage our bodies' cells which is the proof of all disease.

Disease can NOT live, much less thrive in an alkaline environment. Diseases like cancer and kidney disease fade away when you do what this book says to reverse that disease rich acidic state. The huge problem is that even though doctors have no cures and told you there is no cure for your chronic disease, you believed that and will always die because of that deceit.

You have to have the desire to cure yourself. You have to accept the fact that there is a cure for ALL disease outside the medical profession. And you have to get the information to cure yourself and put that information to work for you. This is why I say a lot about attitudes, the way we think and believe in this country. You already know doctors have no cures. So no use even thinking they will cure you. Even when they claim to cure someone, their disease always comes back. That's why they had to make up that nonsense about being a two-time cancer "survivor". They survived cancer but it came back! There is a very obvious reason why it is that way.

Doctors never do a thing about the CAUSE of your diseases! Think about this. Dwell on this absolute Truth! If your water pipe springs a leak, a doctor will just have you mop up the water over and over again. But the rest of us fix the CAUSE of the standing water. That solves the problem with no further service calls or need for a plumber but that one time.

But when it comes to doctors, they refuse to even be interested in you being cured, so they can prolong your illnesses to maximize their incomes. And the solution for that is for YOU to start taking care of your own health so you no longer have to suffer with disease and not be financially drained into having to go bankrupt over excessive medical costs.

So leave your contact with doctors for emergencies and the things doctors actually do, like lab tests, prescribe drugs, surgeries, medical procedures and other lab tests and such. This book is NOT about turning against doctors. This book is about YOU turning to proven science to cure yourselves. **A cure is what saves you from sickness and an early death!** So cures are of paramount importance to those who want to live!

If I had not cured myself, I wouldn't be alive to write this book or any of my other books on cures already available worldwide!

The issue about doctors had to be covered. All of you rely on and trust your doctors with your lives and the lives of your children and other loved ones. That is OK as long as you NEVER EVER believe doctors when they tell you the big lie that your disease cannot be cured.

You will NOT find anything in this book that solves any medical emergencies. You need doctors for ALL serious medical emergencies. Just as your diseases developed over time, all natural cures take time too. You can cure heartburn and dandruff in 3 weeks or so. But those are the exceptions, not the rule for any natural cures.

Once you begin to lay the foundation for your cure, you will know it's working within one to three weeks in almost all cases. Most of you don't really need a doctor for anything while you cure yourselves. But only a rare few people would be willing to do so because of how scared we are when doctors tell us we are going to die real soon.

I never thought I could cure myself. But I did believe doctors would cure me. It was never true. So I had to figure out why I ever thought they would. They wrote in my medical records that I am crazy; because I thought the doctors were going to cure me. And when I started doing the things that eventually cured me, I had no idea I would cure myself or even help myself at all. And when I asked my doctor about taking natural medicines, he said he didn't know a thing about natural medicine. I asked because a lot of vitamins and herb bottles suggest you consult a doctor before taking those items! My doctors wouldn't have anything to do with what I was doing and threw me out of their clinic once they realized I would not be their $100,000 a year dialysis pony.

In spite of that, I do not suggest that anyone should stop seeing their doctors. You can do everything in this book WHILE continuing to follow the advice of your doctors as you choose. Your doctors are either ignorant of the information contained in this book or don't want you to know this information. The sad fact is that it is doctors who should be telling you all of this. But if they do, you will no longer be a source of income for them, or be a source of less income for them. If you're not sick you don't need a doctor.

If you're cured you don't need a doctor. Doctors and hospitals make their money off tests, surgeries, medical procedures and drugs. They don't make money off of you being well, or vitamins, herbs, foods and water. You can patent drugs, but not vitamins and herbs. So it's up to YOU to take care of yourself and it's up to YOU to demand a cure, no matter where it comes from. I was forced to learn these things, as well as forced to experiment on myself, according to the best information I could find and discern as truth, facts or lies in order to have a chance to save my own life.

Doctors said I would be dead or on dialysis by 2008 or 2009 unless I got a successful kidney transplant. It's the beginning of 2013 now. So I assume you can tell I'm not dead? I'm also not on dialysis. But as soon as my doctors in a well-known medical clinic, near our main hospital, realized I was getting better, they sent me certified letters stating that they would no longer be my doctors.

The so-called government is not doing much about the poisons saturating our food, drinks, water and hygiene items. Since it takes regular use of products to kill you, the products are certified "safe" by the FDA. The food companies that make the products and puts all the poisons in them to make you sick, makes billions off you. The medical profession racks in the billions on the diseases those poisons cause. They make billions off you and you are the total loser every step of the way.

But don't waste your time thinking any of these poison peddling billion dollar corporations are going to change or that you could win a lawsuit against any of them. That would take Erin Brockovich! But here's what you can do to take victory over those poisoning you and your families and gain control over your health and hopefully the health of your loved ones too!

And most of you will cure yourself just like I did.

2 - You can afford the cures, not the treatments

I have yet to see more than a rare few who care about their own health. Even as I write this book now, since there is little to no interest by people about actually BEING WELL and BEING CURED, a book like this wouldn't be of value. This book is the best book you could ever read if you want to be cured. Since I wrote my first books on cures, I have had so many people tell me about the results they have gotten.

These results include people reversing their kidney disease, curing diabetes, heartburn, dandruff, heart disease and others; as well as helping many others to recover from traumatic health events like strokes, heart attacks, arthritis headaches and many others.

There is no reason for you to be sick any longer. As I see it, you are only sick because you want to be. OR you haven't done what my books tell you to do to cure yourself

People in this country are affixed to their broken systems. We have a broken government, collapsed economy and a sick care system everyone pretends is a health care system, and that it's the greatest in the world. With over 140 million Americans with at least one chronic disease, I don't know how it could be much more of a failure.

People prefer to spend tens of thousands of dollars for doctors to hold their hands while they lead them to their graves than to take the time to learn to take care of their bodies for pennies on the dollar. One of the main ingredients for every natural cure costs you around $1 a month.

One of my first experiences with doctors about my first chronic disease happened back in the mid-90s when I had several bladder stone attacks. It was back in 1994 I had my first bladder stone attack. I had not been sick or gone to the doctor in about 20 years at that time. I only had one cold during those 20 years. I crawled on the floor screaming in tremendous pain for 4 or 5 days the first two times I had bladder stone attacks. The third time I told my wife that I couldn't take this pain for 4 or 5 days again. So I had her take me to the emergency room. I was there for 6 hours.

When I first got there, I told them I came because I need something for the crippling pain I was suffering. In those 6 hours, they took about a dozen X-rays and finally decided to give me something for my pain! The doctor finally came and told me I needed to check into the hospital for 2-3 days for observation. I argued with him saying that I could not afford, nor did I wish to pay for, a hospital stay. So I told him I was leaving. My bill for those 6 hours was over $1000, and all I got was some pain medication to last a few days.

Once I got the bill, I called the doctor's office, which was right across the street from the hospital. I told them I would pay the outrageous bill as long as they would tell me the cure for bladder stones; since I did not want to keep paying $1000+ each bladder stone attack. Their response was to call me the devil and then threaten to call the police if I didn't stop demanding a cure. I told them "Great. Call the police while you tell me the cure". This just sent the doctor and one of his nurses into a bigger fit.

They continued threatening me while I continued asking them to tell me the cure. None of this got either of us anywhere. And finally, they hung up on me. I told them I was not going to pay the bill unless they told me the cure for bladder stones. As a result, they gave me no cure and I never paid the bill.

Less than a year later, I had my fourth bladder stone attack. I told my wife there was no way I was going back to the emergency room or any damned doctor! As I got to thinking about some things I had learned over the years but never put them to use, I remembered that Magnesium dissolves calcium. Bladder stones, kidney stones and bone spurs are formed by molecules of calcium binding to toxins, free radicals, to form these prickly stones and spurs.

So I took two 250mg Magnesium oxide tablets and in less than an hour, the attack ended. The rest of the day, I peed through a screened filter that I had gotten from the hospital when I went to the ER for my third attack. But no stone was passed. I realized that the Magnesium had dissolved the stone without a visible trace of the stone being left. I began taking 250mg Magnesium oxide every day for a few weeks. Then backed off to taking Magnesium about every other day after that.

I haven't had another bladder stone attack since that day back in 1996. So it's been SEVENTEEN YEARS without another bladder stone attack. Looks like a cure to me!

Believe me, I was shocked about not having another attack. The doctors said I would have bladder stones the rest of my life, since the doctors had NO CURE. So, **it cost me about ten cents to stop my fourth bladder stone attack within an hour;** compared to six hours of x-rays, tests and a $1000+ medical bill and weeks of excruciating pain. Talk about a bargain! As you see, I don't have an opinion. I have the experience and proof about how **you can afford the cures but not the treatments.**

People prefer to eat as much poisons as they choose and never think about what they're doing. They think they can run to the doctor and the doctor will save them from the consequences of their own actions. But what they end up with is one lifelong disease after another and a pile of prescriptions to take every day. You trust your food supply to be safe. You trust your drinks to be safe. You trust your water supplies to be safe. So I've got some advice for you. Stop trusting your food, drinks and water suppliers. What fluoride has to do with safe drinking water is a scam that continues as I write. Don't trust your water company and prove it by getting a water filter to protect yourself.

You can afford a water filter. But you can't afford the medical bills that the chlorine and fluoride will burden you with. Again, it costs about $30-40 a year to prevent brittle bones, bladder cancer and a ravaged immune system; compared to the thousands to tens of thousands of $$$$$ in medical bills for treating the diseases caused by the chlorine and fluoride. You can afford the preventions, but not the treatments.

Like I said - stop trusting your food, drinks and water suppliers. I am not talking about the grocery stores either! The grocery stores put the garbage on the shelves that you buy again and again. If you didn't buy those poison soaked products, they would stop buying those products from their suppliers. Grocery stores stock their shelves with products that sell the fastest. And guess what? For the most part, the healthiest products are the cheapest. If only you were lucky enough to only be able to afford dry beans and brown rice!!!!

The most significant cheap food that is bad for you is white bread. White bread is cheap, but has little to no real nutritional value; whereas whole wheat bread costs 3 times as much, but is highly nutritious. And since bread is a diet staple, you count on eating bread regularly. So it needs to be healthy and nutritious. Otherwise, you get the diseases and conditions white flour causes, starting with chronic diarrhea and intestinal bleeding.

You can afford the cure and prevention, but you can't afford the treatments. The choice is yours to make.

Just remember that it is you that has to make the changes and that it is YOU that can cure yourself. You just need this information so you can!

This table will give you an idea what it will cost you to cure yourself:

Item	One-time costs	Item	Monthly cost
Water filter*	$20* - $110	Baking soda	$1
Shower filter**	$35.00	Vitamin C	$6 - $10
Filter cartridge	$12* - $22** yr.	Fish/Flax seed oil	$8 - $15
		Magnesium	$4.00
Total one-time costs	$55 - $145	Total monthly costs	$19 - $30

So you spend $55-$145 for a shower filter and a charcoal water filter like Water Pik for $55 or $145 for a shower filter and a fluoride water filter. Add to that, $19-$30 monthly for Vitamin C, Flax and/or Fish oil, baking soda and Magnesium and for six months of what you need for the foundation for every cure would be a total cost between $169 to a maximum of around $325. And the next six months would cost you only $114 to $180. Plus the filter replacement cartridges periodically; depending on which filters you get.

Now compare that to your medical bills or just your prescriptions costs and you have the facts about how you can afford the cures but not the costs of medical care for any chronic disease. And besides, this is what a cure costs. Medical costs never include the cost of any cure. They are only for treating your disease and its symptoms and caring for that disease. Cures are affordable. Medical bills are not and neither is the cost of health insurance. You could cure yourself for less than what most people pay for one month's health insurance!

It's facts like these that have caused me to realize how bizarre people think and behave over disease and their worship of doctors as their gods, instead of seeing them as mere men. No matter how great people tell me their doctors are, the one thing they NEVER tell me is that their doctors cured them!

Seek cures, not spite against doctors. Seeking cures is the only one of those things that can help you. To make things a bit clearer about that, I am going to go into a bit more detail about today's medical profession and WHY all of us must cure ourselves IF we are ever to be cured.

After that, I will get to the complete information you need to guide you as you switch from your present "Doctor care sick care" to self-care health care through natural healing.

Summary of "My Cures System"

Now before we go on to cleaning up your current diet I want to explain the perspective, the overall view, of my scientific cures system. All of it is founded on and dictated by proven science. Proven science, the Laws of Science, work the same way 100% of the time. A complete definition of system is "A set of things working together as parts forming a complex whole of a mechanism".

In this case, the mechanism would be cures. So, here are the things you need to be working together as parts of the whole cure for all your diseases. **It doesn't take you conforming to ALL of this to cure you. The more you follow this, the better the results and the quicker those results will come.**

1. **Attitude** – Cures are not a part of today's world. That can only change when your way of thinking changes to include cures as a way of life. Cures are what save you from sickness and an early death. Attitude also includes ending the nonsense about believing FDA approved poisons are safe. Poisons cause 80% of all disease. Over 140 million Americans have chronic diseases because all cures are OUTSIDE the medical profession.

2. **Acidic body state** – You wouldn't be sick unless your body is acidic. So this is why this is the second most important part of my cures system. This is why high pH baking soda is so important. Drink ½-teaspoon baking soda with 4-6 ounces water 2-5x daily for best results. Or eat only fresh fruits and vegetables. Drink Aloe Vera Juice. Use pH drops in your water.

3. **Drink filtered water** – Since your body is 80% water and only a rare few drink proper amounts of water, you have to correct that mistake and drink 1-ounce water for every 2 pounds body weight. Drink water that is filtered through a fluoride filter or a carbon filter according to your budget.

4.   **Shower filter** – Since you soak yourself in chlorinated water and gas in the bath and shower, you need a shower filter. They just screw on your shower water pipe and the shower head screws onto the filter housing. And a shower filter is also the cure for dandruff and itchy dry skin.

5.   **The Perfect Diet** – Basically, pure water and live produce is what I call the perfect diet. If you followed The Perfect Diet, you wouldn't need to use chapters 6 & 7 to clean up your current diet! The Perfect Diet does just that! But only a few would go on The Perfect Diet because of various factors like costs and availability. But The Perfect Diet simplifies the very best diet. The whole Perfect Diet is less than one page. Simple!

6.   **Reading labels to avoid poisons in your food and drinks** – This and #10 are the only complex parts. The foundation of this part is to read labels and avoid all products with the gene mutating poison high fructose corn syrup, high amounts of sugar, salt or fat; as well as white flour, red meat and animal products. Organic milk and eggs, Stevia, raw honey and brown pure cane sugar are not harmful to us. But sugars in liquid drinks do the MOST harm to our bodies. That's how I blew out my kidneys. Watch what you eat & make sure you WATCH WHAT YOU DRINK!

7.   **Vitamin Supplementation** - To correct rampant deficiencies in the American diet. - No one is able to stay healthy because of the low amounts of nutrients in our food supplies due to the endless chemicals burning farm lands and saturating the soil plants grow in. So supplement your diet to at least correct the major deficiencies we all have. Those include Vitamin C, Magnesium and Omega-3. But your body needs all nutrients you can think of and more. So learn to add things to your diet that will give you those nutrients. And use vitamin supplementation to insure that you are getting enough of those nutrients.

8.   **Take Herbs** – Herbs are natural plant medicines and the only medicines man had until the infusion of synthetic toxic chemical medicines totally replaced our natural herbal medicines. You need to remember this major fact too. All herbal medicines are safe and were used by mankind since the first man lived on this earth. But all the synthetic chemical medicines used today have only been used 70 years or less. Rational thinking leads us to use herbs, while the mindless choice we all make is to trust all these drugs that haven't existed very long. Stupid, huh! Herbs were also the foundation of the practice of Hippocrates', the Father of Medicine, along with fasting. The herbs you should consider first are Lemon Balm, Sage, Astragalus, Bilberry, Garlic, Cayenne, Turmeric and Hawthorn Berries.

9.   **Fasting – Fasting forces your body to use its energy to heal your body and repair damaged cells instead of for digesting food.** All other energy is used for body metabolisms and removing toxins. Fasting 12-16 hours often is easier than trying to go days without food. The idea

is to cut down on ingesting anything with calories so that energy is used for healing you. You can't correct nutrient deficiencies by fasting though. To fast for days, try taking your Vitamin C, Omega-3 and Magnesium with water while eating one piece of fruit like an apple or orange. Never fast without drinking plenty of water. If you are near death, don't fast until you have been doing the things listed before fasting, so you can nourish your body back to health a bit before putting stress on it fasting.

10. **Grocery shopping attitude** – The grocery store is the front line in your change for the better. That is where you get all those poisons saturated foods and drinks. If you read labels in the grocery store, you won't even buy those products to be ABLE to consume them at home. You have to become the guardian of your food and drinks. I am an expert and I can't tell you more than a few products that are NOT bad for you. So this is one of the toughest ones. You just gotta settle yourself on taking the time to read the labels and not put the bad ones in your basket! Try reading chapters 6 and 7 right before you do your grocery shopping. That way you'll have those facts fresh in your mind when you go. And be VERY proud of yourself that you are making the effort to save you and your family from sickness, suffering and an early death.

11. **Exercise** – Although I don't know of any disease that is caused by lack of exercise, exercise is still helpful in improving your health. You need to get your heart pumping faster than normal, naturally. Exercise does just that. Exercise speeds up your metabolism. When you're sick, it speeds up your sickness. When you are curing yourself, exercise speeds up your healing cures and makes your body stronger.

Fasting is really more important than its order in this list, because your body heals itself. Your body naturally works to repair damaged cells and heal your body until it is forced to divert its energy for digesting food. THE thing you want to do is get your body healing itself as much as is possible. You just have to find a safe compromise between fasting for healing and diverting healing energy for digestion. Cutting down on the amount of food you eat will help a lot.

So do that, and fast for 12-16 hours often. And when you think you can do it, fast for a whole day or 2 or 3 at a time. Making your body heal you 24 hours a day is far better for you than the 15 hours or more your body spends digesting food. That means that only 9 hours does your body have a chance to use its energy for healing. And the #1 thing you need is healing power! So **fasting could very well belong after attitude as far as its value in curing you.**

These 11 parts constitute my system to cure all disease. My entire system of cures depends on you every step of the way! It saves your life and your money!

Other than these 11 things, all you need is a doctor for lab tests and a few prescriptions. So let's get on to the rest of the information you need to guide you away from the saturation of poisons in our food, drinks and water supplies.

3 - The Modern Medical Profession's Sick Care System

As for the modern medical profession in this country.....

To sum it up in as few words as possible, the modern medical profession in the USA is among the very best in the world in emergency situations and among the very worst in the world at curing disease.

If you have a car wreck or a traumatic accident or injury, be glad that you live in this country. But if you want to be cured of your diseases, you live in one of the very worst countries. You don't hear this in the media or government. All they ever tell us is how we have the greatest health care in the world. They don't want to talk about the near 1,000,000 people a year that have to file bankruptcy because of grossly inflated medical bills.

They don't want to talk about the 50,000,000 Americans that don't have any health care. They don't want to talk about the 25,000 Americans who die as a direct cause of FDA certified "safe" prescription drugs yearly. They don't want to talk about the 100,000 Americans that die each year because of medical procedures. They don't want to talk about how we cannot continue paying these huge medical bills as individuals or a nation.

And what else don't they want to talk about? They don't want to talk about natural cures or preventing disease, much less, talk about the saturation of poisons in our food, drinks and water that are causing almost all sickness and disease. And until they START, there is no hope of these problems being solved by them. As a result, we have many plagues of chronic disease.

Here are some startling facts about chronic disease in America as proof.

Chronic Diseases are the Leading Causes of Death & Disability in the USA

- 7 out of 10 deaths among Americans each year are from chronic diseases. Heart disease, cancer and stroke account for more than 50% of all deaths each year.
- In 2005, 133 million Americans – almost 1 out of every 2 adults – had at least one chronic illness.
- Obesity has become a major health concern. 1 in every 3 adults is obese and almost 1 in 5 youth between the ages of 6 and 19 is obese (BMI $\geq$ 95th percentile of the CDC growth chart).
- About one-fourth of people with chronic conditions have one or more daily activity limitations.
- Arthritis is the most common cause of disability, with nearly 19 million Americans reporting activity limitations.
- Diabetes continues to be the leading cause of kidney failure, nontraumatic lower-extremity amputations, and blindness among adults, aged 20-74,

Now, with 133,000,000 Americans in 2005 who have at least one chronic disease, is that what you call the result of the best health care system in the world? Yes you do! But it's complete nonsense. Each of those 133,000,000 Americans represents a failure of this country's medical profession. Even with 10,000,000 Americans with chronic disease, we should have declared a national emergency. But with 133,000,000 Americans with at least one chronic disease, we not only haven't declared a national emergency, we continue to declare that we have the best health care on the planet! If every single person had at least one chronic disease, they would still tell you that and you would still believe them! I don't know of any greater incompetence in any profession or line of work than this country's medical profession and health care system.

When I got the statistics above from the <u>Center for Disease Control web site</u>, I noticed their web site also talked about what causes these chronic diseases. But guess what they did NOT mention in that information? Not one word about poisons in your food, drinks and water supplies. The closest they came was naming cigarettes or alcohol as a cause of lung cancer or liver disease. Whoop dee Do! But it's the same thing at the doctor's office!

Rarely does a doctor tell you what caused your chronic disease. I have asked almost everyone I have talked to, if their doctor has ever told them what caused their chronic disease. I never get any specific answers, just vague generalizations! Now that's what you should be getting from rank amateurs, but NOT from professionals! A professional is assumed to be an expert in their field or occupation. But how can you call the medical profession that has failed to cure the diseases of over 133,000,000 people at this very moment, "experts"! Face reality as it is! With over 133,000,000 known cases of complete failure by this country's doctors and medical profession, it's well past time to try something new. You know - something that does NOT have over 133,000,000 known failures at any given moment! And near 150 million here in 2013.

With that huge amount of documented failures by the modern medical profession, you would think they would be bursting at the seams to find cures for all of that sickness and disease. Look at all that research they do and how many billions of dollars go into that research. Isn't it wonderful that this goes on in this county! I mean, to have these guys taking your donations and doing that incredibly hard and intense research to uh.......... research some more, then .....uh, research even more.......then, uh.......... let's keep on researching ....and uh..... never find a cure! Hey, if you find a cure, then your RESEARCH won't be needed any more! Whoops!

It's the same thing at the doctor's office too. Now why would they cure you just so they could lose your business? They wouldn't and that's the main reason they don't.

It's like I said earlier in this book about what happened at the ER and with the doctor who attended me in the ER. I asked them to give me the cure for bladder stones, and they not only couldn't or wouldn't tell me, they called me the devil and threatened to call the police on me. I just told them "OK, I'm the devil and you're calling the police on me. But could you just give me the cure for bladder stones?" I never got that cure from them. They only told me about how I would have bladder stones the rest of my life, and that they were "incurable". They tried to talk me into a few days stay in the hospital, instead of telling me the cure in the first place!!!!! The doctor was just being a businessman making the sales pitch for his services, and I was only his customer.

Same thing when they threw me out of Clopton Clinic. They only offered death and dialysis within 2-3 years. But I only cared about being cured. My failure to submit to them and throw away my life caused my two doctors to lose interest in me; since I was not going to be their $100,000 a year dialysis pony. Remember, those doctors never had a second of interest in finding out what I was doing to achieve what they had never achieved; even though THEY are the so-called "experts" and professionals in this!

They made it crystal clear to me that curing people is not something they are interested in. I thought they were just picking on ME at the time, but I haven't found any cures in the medical profession. It's not isolated to these two doctors and one clinic in this one town! The fact that over 133,000,000 Americans have diseases doctors have no cures for backs that up.

You have to understand that our pathetic system forces individuals to go to college for 8 years, then Medical school for at least 4-6 years to become a doctor. Then you have an intern-ship before you are an official doctor. That costs several $100,000! These individuals are entitled to recoup these expenses and earn a decent living. But the inherent problems of this system forces doctors to become businessmen in order to be a doctor.

Please don't think I'm suggesting you make any effort to fix this. I'm not. They need to fix their own system. We, the People need to do what it takes to prevent and cure our own sickness and disease and not make any medical services depend on MONEY! But there's another side to it. We need to take responsibility as individuals and work on eliminating the poisons from our food, drinks and water supplies to prevent disease from occurring in the first place.

Doctors and medical facilities invest huge sums of money in technology and have to get money from you to pay for all that technology. That technology is used to diagnose diseases and conditions. So, it's invaluable to both them and you. When I first went to the doctor about my kidneys, they said I had to have two CAT scans to check for kidney stones. When the doctor told me that, I blurted out "I couldn't have kidney stones. I take Magnesium regularly." The look on the doctor's face was that same look you'd get if you said something like "I'm going to beat up your mother!" LOL I got the same look about 2 months later when I slipped and told the same doctor how drinking lemon balm tea had stopped the blood and blood clots in my piss. He snapped at me immediately and yelled "Well, did your lemon balm tea tell you you have chronic kidney disease?"

Now if I hadn't known that kidney stones, bladder stones and bone spurs were not possible, since it is lack of Magnesium that allows these "calcium deposits" to form in the first place, I would have thrown away $1100. Not to mention, the $1000 this scientific fact had already saved me by curing me of bladder stones, and the thousands more I saved by not needing medical attention for future bladder stone attacks. If the doctors are so sure you need those tests, then why don't they ever agree to pay for those tests if they're wrong? DUH! But we all know it's you that has to pay for those unnecessary tests. What you are not understanding is that the medical profession makes its money off YOUR sickness, disease and conditions. What they offer is:

Examinations, tests, drugs, surgeries and medical procedures taught in Medical schools. So if you need these services you go to the doctor and medical professionals. And IF you can get a cure from the doctor, then you want it, right? But most of the "cures" I hear from the medical profession are followed by the same diseases coming right back within a very few years.

It's because the doctors never care what caused the disease in the first place. They are just there to treat your disease and give you medical attention and services. They are not trained or licensed to counsel or aid you in making a diet or lifestyle change. Doctors also aren't allowed to use herbs or any natural cures to help you. Their solutions are ONLY what Medical schools teach them to do: examinations, tests, drugs, surgeries and medical procedures taught in Medical schools.

The medical profession began to race into greed and away from real health care in the 1940's. That was when the first patented drug was mass produced; which was penicillin. Since then, drug companies have turned their interests to man-made drugs so they can patent them and mass-produce them. It seems that drug companies run this country. And in the past 20 years, technology has become the core of the medical industry. We're paying out the nose for that technology. And does any of that technology cure anyone? Are any of those patented drugs curing anyone? If they are, then why are you still taking those drugs! And guess what? Your body bears the evidence that these drugs are not good for you.

The minute any drug goes into your body, your system starts to work to remove all those drugs. That's why you have to keep taking them. Your body doesn't use any of those drugs. So nature itself bears the proof that drugs are not good for you. I am not telling you to cease taking your medications. I am telling you about a better way of naturally curing yourself that requires you to face the facts as they are. All this points to "There's got to be a better way." And there is. As people grow older they go from ONE drug to THREE drugs, to FIVE drugs, to EIGHT drugs, then on to TEN or TWELEVE drugs. And regardless of what temporary good they do, they are all still poisons your body works to remove as soon as you take them.

And to protect the drug companies' monopolies on drug sales, our Treasonous government continues their fascist and completely UN-Constitutional war against the People in the name of drugs. Hundreds and hundreds of billions of your taxpayer dollars are spent on this illegal drug war to protect these drug companies' drug dealing monopolies. That, along with hundreds of billions more taxpayer dollars to pay to imprison those who don't buy their drugs from these drug companies.

Just as the entire medical profession abandoned all cures in the 1940's after the first chemical drug was patented, the so-called government began its campaign against natural plant medicines with its baseless propaganda about marijuana. That is how our nation's #1 medicine was taken away from The People. That illegal "drug war" continues to this day and is the major source of systematic violations of civil rights by a lawless fascist government that refuses to acknowledge the basic self-evident Truth that we are endowed by our Creator with the Right to make our own personal choices, regardless of who does not agree with those personal choices.

I know adults have the Right to make their own choices. And the only thing criminal Laws are for, is to protect us all from abuse by others; NOT to protect us from our own choices. But these are the facts about how our government has used our own tax money to attempt to wipe out our nation's #1 medicine while they ignore and fight AGAINST all natural medicines man ever used. And that repulsive behavior is why doctors have NO cures and do not practice real medicine at all. They don't even acknowledge any natural medicines, even though the only medicines this planet had until 1940 was nothing BUT natural plant medicines, herbs, like our former #1 natural medicine marijuana!

Their war against the People in the name of drugs is a huge failure and was never about illegal drugs. It was always about controlling people and squashing basic Civil Rights under the US Constitution and Bill of Rights; and to go after anyone who was cutting into corporate drug companies' sales and profits.

Possession of drugs is a crime against yourself. Problem with that is that you can NOT commit a crime against yourself under the US Constitution. Criminal Laws are written to protect individuals from being harmed by others. I have the Right to choose to do illegal drugs, just as I have the Right to choose to do legal drugs. I believe in and live by the US Constitution and Bill of Rights. Those protect MY freedom, not any man, soldiers or government.

The war on drugs has to end or shift its focus to the 25,000 – 100,000 people who die from prescription drugs each year, instead of pouring tens of billions of dollars into going after illegal drugs that only kill around 4,000 people each year in this country. Their drug war has been a main factor in the destruction of America, and all because American citizens choose to get their drugs from other sources besides doctors and pharmacies; who by the way, sell the drugs made by the drug corporations.

As a result, our prisons are filled with those who made individual choices for themselves about who they get THEIR drugs from, while nothing ever happens to the doctors whose drugs kill tens of thousands of people each year. I am not suggesting we prosecute every doctor. It's the total immunity from prosecution for doctors that never was legal. In this country, it's never the ACT that determines if a crime has been committed. They always have to know WHO it was that committed the crime before they admit it's a crime.

You should check your US Constitution and you will clearly see that the US Constitution does two major things. It confirms and establishes by Supreme Law that Individual Rights are the Supreme authority of the United States, and establishes government with specific and limited Rights. Fascism rules over this country by exalting the imaginary UN-Constitutional Rights of government, corporations, churches, lobbyists and other groups above Individual Rights.

You have the Right to say anything you want to say, unless your government doesn't agree with what you say. Then you go jail. UN-Constitutional "laws" are the rule in this treasonous democracy, not the exception. America is a Republic, not a democracy.

One of the newest betrayals of Public Trust is states passing blatant anti-Constitutional bills requiring all those receiving government assistance to take drug tests. The Constitution prohibits government from conducting illegal searches and seizures saying "The Right of the People to be secure in their persons, papers, houses and effects against unreasonable searches and seizures shall not be violated.........." except with a warrant, naming the places to be searched and the things to be seized.

Now if the government wants to drug test you legally, they will have to first have reasonable cause that you are doing illegal drugs. Seizing your blood and searching it without reasonable cause AND a search warrant is UN-Constitutional and therefore supremely illegal! I hope you refuse to take the drug test if your state stoops as low as Florida already has.

If I had it MY way, doctors would be taught, then required to CURE their patients and never talk about a person NOT being cured of any chronic disease. The simplest way of saying that is, if doctors would start curing us with proven science, rare few people would ever need a book like this to cure their diseases. But since doctors never cure anyone, ALL those cures are only found OUTSIDE the modern medical profession.

I do want to say that I am not going into the politics about the health care reform bill, the outrageous $500 billion Medicare drug bill Congress passed a few years back, health care fraud or anything like that. I believe every human deserves food, shelter, clothing and medical care. But in this country, you either pay for it or you do without these basic human Rights. But if you prevent most disease in the first place, you won't need doctors and medical bills very much at all. And that's what they are really warring against – We, the People not being poisoned to death by corporations through our food, drinks and water. AND..... as a result of that aggressive poisoning, we turn to doctors who treat us and care for our endless diseases, but NEVER EVER cure them!

Preventing disease can save up to 80% of all medical bills, and that includes Medicaid and Medicare. That's why I **see Preventative medicine as the only TRUE health care reform.**

You know that Congress is never going to go along with anything that cuts the profits or decreases business for the insurance and medical industries. Right now, all we have is a fascist tyranny that exalts the imaginary Rights of corporations, government and other groups above the Rights of Individuals.

Now, back to the medical profession and one of its biggest problems concerning you. Has your doctor ever taken your blood pressure correctly? Did they follow these rules when taking your blood pressure?

- Maintain proper posture - Sit in a chair with your:
- Back supported - Legs uncrossed - Feet flat on the floor
- Rest and relax
- Sit and relax for 5 minutes before taking your blood pressure.
- Do not talk while you are taking you're blood pressure.
- Wait one full minute between multiple measurements.
- Wait at least 30 minutes after any nicotine, caffeine, alcohol, other stimulants or meals.
- Wait at least 60 minutes after any strenuous exercise.

Well did you know that the scale used for determining normal blood pressure and all stages of hypertension only apply IF these rules are followed? I have never had my blood pressure taken by any doctor following these rules. One time a male nurse was kind enough to follow these rules at my request, and my blood pressure was the lowest it ever was at the doctor's office. If you have the same experience at the doctor's office that I do, they make you wait 30 minutes after your appointed time and that makes you tense, anxious. Then they take you to a room, sit you down and take your blood pressure.

So, don't ever give any credibility to blood pressure readings at the doctor's office. Your blood pressure goes up when you eat, exercise, talk and for pretty much everything you do. But it's NORMAL. So you have to take your blood pressure when you're relaxed inside and out, or the scale doesn't matter.

I use to take my blood pressure 30-40 times a day to see what my blood pressure was under all kinds of circumstances. My blood pressure was always high unless I followed the rules above. Lots of times I would take my blood pressure as soon as I sat down. Then I would take my blood pressure 4 more times. Each reading would go down a little more than the last. The difference between my first and last reading averaged about 40/25. Doctors are SUPPOSE to be the experts on blood pressure. But my experiences with the medical profession have only shown me that they are not experts about blood pressure. They either don't know the rules or don't care. They care as little about correct blood pressure as they do cures.

Now, I COULD go on about more problems with the medical profession. But talking about their problems won't really cure you or prevent any diseases. You need information about that. But I had to talk about some of the major things about the modern medical profession in this country to help you put things in the proper perspective. **No matter how wrong you know something is, it doesn't solve any problems. You need solutions.**

And with over 133,000,000 documented failures existing at all times with the medical profession, it's way past time to face up to this massive incompetence and speak up and out for what you need - cures for all your diseases. That is what this book is about and helps YOU to accomplish for yourselves. And you can do so WHILE you listen to your doctors, except for the parts about death and there's no cure.

Rarely will a doctor agree to be a part of anyone curing themselves. But pretending your doctors might help you, will keep most of you from being afraid while you cure yourselves naturally. It does terrify you when the doctors tell you that you have one of those diseases that will kill you if you only listen to doctors.

Oh how I wish I had this book when I was first diagnosed with chronic kidney disease! Oh how I wish I knew the things in this book BEFORE I was diagnosed with CKD. I knew about eating right. I just didn't know about drinking right too, or how saturated with poisons our entire food and drinks supplies really are.

I didn't want to get into politics, religion or anything that would divert your attention to it, and therefore distract you from the facts you need to eliminate poisons so that you can be cured. You don't need to call your Congressman, doctor, grocery store, food corporations or anyone. You need to get to work protecting you and your family from this saturation of poisons in your food, drinks, water supplies and hygiene items. There was no use in going over how many people have unnecessary surgeries and dwell on that either. But it is funny how when doctors cut you open and remove things out of your body, you pay them large sums of money and praise them. But if a stranger cuts you open on the street, you would file criminal charges and curse them to Hell and back.

That's just a clear sign of how this country has no morals. It depends on who commits the act. The same action by a doctor is wrong when some who is not a doctor does the same thing. Just as no matter how many crimes police officers commit, it's never a crime because of who they are. Our Nation's problem could be solved IF the US Constitution ever becomes valid Law again some day. Then, We the People would be the government; organized to help We the People. And food, shelter, clothing and health care would be human Rights. That means you qualify for health care by being human!

But just as the medical profession has no cures for the chronic diseases of over 133,000,000 Americans, the phony government has a debt crisis, collapsed economy, widespread unbridled greed, a failed 40 year drug war, occupies over 150 foreign countries militarily, still fighting two worthless wars, 50 million people without health care, millions homeless., the largest prison population on the planet and no end or solutions in sight. This nation stills expects different results and consequences from the same actions. But that has never happened and never will. This country use to be great when its citizens had Rights. Empowering individuals is what can make a country great. You have heard that knowledge is Power, and that is true. The knowledge in this book empowers each individual to take control of their health and get your lives back. Going to the empty hole for cures is never going to help.

Don't you assume that you are going to the doctor to be cured? Don't you assume the doctor will tell you what will help you? Don't you assume that your doctor can be trusted to do what is best for you? Well, none of this is true, and it's up to you to face the facts as they are. When I point out how doctors want you to be sick and stay sick to maximize their income or other absolute facts about doctors, they almost always tell me "My doctor's not like that. He 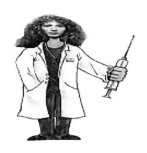 really cares about me." Chuckle, chuckle chuckle....is all I can ever reply!

Oh and, uh hey, if your doctor really cared, why didn't he cure you? But even though your doctor did not cure you, you still go along with what he says and keep going back. This makes no sense whatsoever! If you lose your car keys, what do you do - look on the TV, and if they're not there you never drive again? No you don't! You keep looking for those keys until you find them and you know it! But when it comes to your own life and health, you go along with the doctors, never get a cure, and never look elsewhere for a cure.

Sure, you might get a second or third doctor's opinion. But you don't look elsewhere, outside the medical profession. And **that's where all the cures are - outside the medical profession. So go to your doctors and get your cures OR LOOK ELSEWHERE for your cures. In other words, start acting normal about your health and life.**

We're all being poisoned to death through our food, drinks, water supplies and hygiene items. The food corporations make billions of dollars off the addictive poisons they saturate our food, drinks and hygiene supplies with; which creates up to 80% of the business for the medical industry, who also makes billions of dollars off your pain and suffering. And they do so with the phony government doing little to nothing to protect us from any of this. And every step of the way YOU ARE THE LOSER! You pay your money for the poisons, then pay for help with the medical problems those poisons cause you.

And none of this is really your fault.

You could blame yourself, but you didn't put those poisons in any of those things. So, **why do we have to suffer the consequences for the poisons THEY put in our food, drinks and water that the government declares "safe"? I will tell you exactly why you have to suffer the consequences for THEIR wrongs. You made one big mistake!!!!!!!! What was that one big mistake? You were born in this country! That's the huge mistake you made in all this! If you hadn't been born in this country, you wouldn't be suffering and losing your lives because of the saturation of poisons the food and drinks corporations are putting in those products.**

So the solution is obvious. Don't anyone else be born in this country! Silly, right! Of course. All you can do is read this book as a guide to avoiding these poisons in our food, drinks and water supplies. You have to understand that as long as the solution to your problem depends on you, there is nothing but hope. But if your solution depends on food corporations, government, doctors, the medical profession or anyone else, there's no real hope for any solutions.

And by the way, I originally titled this book "Murdered by America" because of the facts I just stated. But I wasn't technically murdered by America. I was almost murdered by this country and its ways and systems. But this country doesn't even resemble America anymore; mostly for the reasons I pointed out earlier. The U.S. Constitution is the proof of that. And our food, drinks and water supplies are only the delivery devices for their poisons. So it's all up to you as individuals to empower yourselves through knowledge, and the Power of this book will guide you as you climb that mountain that stands between you and your well-being. The government, medical profession and corporations have indeed established themselves as obstacles to our freedom, peace and well-being; rather than the source of our solutions to those unalienable Rights.

But hey, our nation was great when Individual Rights were protected. And the only hope I have for this Nation is IF and WHEN our Individual Rights are taken back by each individual, and the US Constitution is once again the Supreme Law of the Land. It's been many many years since I heard "Our nation is only as strong as the weakest citizens in the nation." We never hear that anymore because if we say that, then we know our Nation is weak, helpless, homeless, immoral, violent, poor, sick and without any freedom. So we never hear that any more. But I say - bring that saying back.

It's that great American spirit that can solve all these problems, as long as We, the People means every American citizen, instead of We, the Corporations as it is now.

The U.S. Health care system is ranked #1 in cost of care by the WHO, World Health Organization. But.......

The U.S. Health care system is ranked #37 in the quality of that most expensive care in the entire world.

4 - Things to Do As the Foundation for Every Cure

There are things you need to do for any and every cure. And with some of you, just one of these things could cure you and save your life. A good example of this is cancer. Baking soda water will cure cancer. Taking 5,000-10,000mg of Vitamin C daily will cure cancer. And eating hardly anything but fresh fruits and vegetable will cure cancer. Do all three and the cure for your cancer is certain. But to maintain your cure you must deal with the cause of your disease, which is poisons; most of which are in our food, drinks and water supplies.

Becoming a vegetarian can save your life. But being a vegetarian does not eliminate all the poisons that cause almost all disease. This is why I have to stay founded on the principles which deal with the cause of disease and not get into thinking that everyone will become a vegetarian by reading this book and not eat anything BUT fresh fruits and vegetables. So what I am doing is telling you how to gracefully and naturally change your ways so that you are no longer blind and naïve to the reality of what you put into your body by trusting your food, drinks and water supplies and those who provide those things.

If we had a government, We the People would not allow food and drink corporations to poison us and addict us to their imitation food products. Most of our foods and drinks are nothing but the drugs white flour, sugar and the bad poison known as high fructose corn syrup, aka HFCS. HFCS is made with genetically altered corn using genetically altered enzymes; making it a GMO. A GMO is a Genetically Modified Organism. And just imagine what something as viciously poisonous as HFCS does once it gets inside your cancer-ridden body or any chronically diseased body. Do you really wonder WHY you are sick!

Although this is the worst poison, it is only part of the problem about how our American diet is killing us all, while the medical profession prolongs our diseases those those poison products caused. There are rare few products at the grocery store that are not saturated with disease causing poisons. So even though our goal is to not get sick, we've gained this attitude that we will eat what we want to, then just let doctors save us from what we did to ourselves.

Regardless of this gross irresponsibility, this is normal behavior in this nation. Yes, you can choose to eat anything you want. But your choice can never change science. So since science is not going to change, either YOU have to change, OR suffer and die! The real problem is with the absence of any real government, these poisons are allowed in the products we consume. HFCS should never have been allowed. PERIOD.

But as long as you are peddling these disease causing poisons, that is what they should be called. And they should NOT be allowed to call those products food products. At least require them to label those products like Twinkies, Coke, Pepsi, Oreos and all the ones like those to be labeled as Imitation food, synthetic food or similar. And also require warning labels on those products about the diseases that regular use of those products WILL cause.

But since we do not have a government to do those things, it is up to each and every one of us to learn to recognize those poisons and avoid them. That's why what I teach is based on the three chapters Poisons in Your Water, Drinks and Food. It is those chapters that guide you in cleaning up the American diet of acidic red meat and acidic sugars. It is sugars, white flour and animal products that make our bodies acidic so that disease can form and thrive. And since our food supplies are so low in nutrients due to the chemicals that have leeched and made barren the very soil almost all food is grown in, the American diet has built-in major nutrient deficiencies.

It is those problems that we have to recognize and take steps to correct. And it is those problems that I will tell you the solutions to now. So let's take the first and most important problem first. That problem is the acidic condition we ate and drank our bodies into that allowed disease to form in our bodies at all. So the first step in any and every cure is to correct the acidic state of our body.

There are several ways to correct that acidic state. The best way by far is to drink baking soda water two or more times daily. One half teaspoon baking soda mixed in 4-6 ounces of the purest water you can afford. This flushes your kidneys with highly alkaline water. Those with kidney disease reverse the metabolic acidosis that causes almost all kidney disease. It also dissolves Uric acid kidney stones.

Your kidneys regulate what the contents of your blood are. So as that baking soda water flushes your kidneys, that causes your kidneys to produce blood that is more alkaline. And as that increasingly more alkaline blood flows through your body, it neutralizes acidity throughout your entire body! As a result, your diseases can no longer exist; and fade away naturally. It is this proven science that makes this the most important thing to do to cure yourself.

Other highly alkaline things you can put in your body to help reverse and neutralize acid in your body is Aloe Vera Juice. Drinking Aloe Vera juice can help a lot, but not as well as drinking the baking soda water. The same is true about pH drops you can add to your drinking water. Using pH drops helps a lot too. I used pH drops until I had the proof about baking soda. And of course, just eating fresh fruits and vegetables will help reverse the acidic state of your body.

Do not underestimate the power of baking soda. There are so many things you can use baking soda for. Using it to reverse the acidic state of your body is just one use. I'll tell you some more uses later on. **One caution about baking soda is that those who have high blood pressure should not drink baking soda water if your high blood pressure is caused by excessive salt in your blood. I only recommend drinking baking soda to cure disease. So drink it only on occasion if you are not sick or have high blood pressure from excessive salt in your blood.** But for now, let's move on to the next part of the foundation for any cure – nutrient deficiencies.

There is no way you COULD get enough nutrients, minerals and enzymes to stay healthy just by eating what you buy at the grocery store. So you have to take vitamins and herbs to have a chance to stay healthy in this backwards third world nation this country has become. Remember, this is the only "civilized" nation that does NOT provide health-care for all its citizens. But the fact is, this fact alone confirms that this nation is NOT a civilized nation! So it's up to each of us to save ourselves from the monsters that poison us to death and the monsters that refuse to cure us and will only TREAT and CARE for our diseases.

So with baking soda as the most important thing in reversing our diseases and curing us, what are the major diet deficiencies in the American diet and what can we do to correct those diet deficiencies?

You need to take Vitamin C, Fish oil and flax seed oil and magnesium. Vitamin C is deficient in our diets, but since our bodies do not make or store Vitamin C we have to take supplements to get enough Vitamin C to keep us healthy and free of disease. Take 1000mg Vitamin C if you don't have any disease and take anywhere from 3000-10,000mg daily if you do have diseases. I have provided a chart in a later chapter showing you the recommended dosages for certain diseases. But what is Vitamin C going to do to cure me?

Vitamin C is a readily available anti-oxidant. Anti-oxidants remove the toxins, poisons and free radicals that cause all disease in our bodies. You need Vitamin C and other anti-oxidants to remove those toxins to keep your diseases from getting any worse. If toxins are being removed, then they can't damage the nucleus of cells to create cancer cells, for example. So take Vitamin C and as many other anti-oxidants as you choose, such as Vitamin A and E, Selenium, Alpha Lipoic Acid and others.

Next is magnesium. Without enough Magnesium over 300 body metabolisms do not occur. This is the same thing that happens as your body gets more and more acidic by consuming sugars and animal products. So merely taking 400mg of Magnesium daily, those 300+ body metabolisms begin taking place once again in your body. And you sure can't say where you are getting enough Magnesium in your diet. So vitamin supplementation of Magnesium is a must if you expect to cure yourself and stay cured.

Then, add to that about 2000-5000mg Fish oil and/or flax seed oil to provide the Omega-3 the savage American diet could never give you and you have the basic foundation for EVERY cure! The lack of Omega-3 in your diet results in diseases like arthritis, Alzheimer's, strokes, heart attacks, Parkinson's and other brain diseases. Omega-3 also reduces the inflammation that accompanies all diseases. If man was on the fish diet man is suppose to be on, an Omega-3 deficiency would not occur. But with the red meat and sugar American diet, there is no way anyone could not have an Omega-3 deficiency, Magnesium deficiency and Vitamin C deficiency.

To sum all this up, here is what you need to lay the foundation for every cure:

- Baking soda water - ½ teaspoon with 4-6 oz. Water 2-5x daily
- Vitamin C – 3,000 – 10,000mg daily depending on the disease
- Magnesium oxide – 400-800mg daily for 4-6 weeks, then 400mg daily
- Omega-3 – 2000-5000mg fish or flax seed oil daily

This sums up what you need to start with. I explained why this is the foundation for every cure. Later on in the chapter MORE Cures and Preventions, I give you more things you can do for certain diseases to speed your cure along. But the baking soda water, Vitamin C, Magnesium and Omega-3 are the foundation for every cure. Drinking as much clean filtered water as you can is also a major part of every cure.

You need water to flush the toxins out of your body and to replace all that acidic chlorinated water you have consumed since birth. I do not recommend drinking lots of non-filtered water, since your body has to remove all that chlorine, fluoride and other poisons in all our water supplies. That $20 for a charcoal filter, $110 for a fluoride filter or hundreds of dollars for an osmosis filter or better, is an investment in your health that provides great benefits. You need to drink 1 ounce of water for every 2 pounds body weight daily. The value of pure clean water is so important that the main part of your cures depends on water. This is why the next chapter is about Poisons in Your Water.

And as I explain all throughout this book and all my books, changing your way of thinking, attitude adjustments, is part of the foundation for every cure. In this backwards third world nation, cures are never talked about! Cures aren't even mentioned in this country except on the rarest of occasions. So how can you ever expect to be cured as long as you never talk about cures? So the first thing you need to do is start talking about cures.

I know that when I talk about cures on places like Facebook, it's as though I posted something in a foreign language! People don't know what to say since cures are not a part of this country's medical profession, government, religious institutions or among the people. Cures are what saves you from sickness and death. So cures are of the most paramount importance. And since the helpless fascist media in this country only reports what doctors do, we never hear a peep about cures from them. It's the entire Media too.

I even asked our local TV station and newspaper to help spread the word about cures to save lives. But they were bigots about it. After KAIT-TV refused to inform little children with cancer about the cure for cancer recently, they even ran a story a few weeks later about a FAKE cure some doctor in the state of Mississippi claimed about curing a baby with AIDS. As it turns out, the baby NEVER even had AIDS! But KAIT-TV rushed to report this fraud because they are intolerant of We the People. Same is true with the Jonesboro Sun. They'll report how doctors cured someone. Then a few weeks of months later they run a story telling us how these people that "doctors cured" have died! And this vulgar fascist deceit is never going to end with the media!

So when you make the choice to cure yourself, no one is going to help you except YOU and proven science like this book provides you with. But the great thing is that you get cured and don't go bankrupt paying the medical bills to those who never cure anyone and don't even have an interest in cures.

So along with the baking soda, magnesium, anti-oxidants, Omega-3 and water, you need attitude adjustments and changing your current ways that made you sick in the first place.

But in this savage third world nation, most everyone is addicted to the huge amounts of poisons in our food and drinks. So you have to deal with those addictions that are in your mind. Those addictions are real and very serious. It has been proven that sugar and especially high fructose corn syrup cause a change in the chemistry of your brain identical to what drugs like cocaine and meth-amphetamine cause in your brain.

Fructose is a natural sugar found in all fruits. Loving the fruit and the natural fructose in fruit is what food and drink corporations have focused on to addict you to their poisonous imitation food products, They make you a robot zombie that consumes their products mindlessly! Only in the food and drink corporations are they allowed to deliberately addict you to the drugs in their products. There is nothing right or legal about any of it either. Only through the deep-seated corruption of the FDA and other government agencies is this massive drugging of the people allowed!

And since they are never going to stop this heinous behavior, all you CAN do is learn to read all labels and avoid as much of those deadly poisons as you can. And since this entire greedy nation suffers like this, the main focus of this book is to teach you how to clean up your current diet. Doing that is far more practical than telling you that you have to become a vegetarian if you ever want to be cured. This is why the next chapters are Poisons in Your Water, Poisons in Your Drinks and Poisons in Your Food.

If you can do it, stick with becoming a vegetarian as the simplest way of curing yourself and restoring your body to a disease free state. If you want the simplest information about proper diet, try following what I call The Perfect Diet.

The Perfect Diet....

What do I mean by The Perfect Diet? If I could eat the healthiest diet of food and drinks, what would that diet consist of? Right off you would say eat fresh fruits and vegetables ONLY and drink pure water The problem you would have is that there are poisons inside all produce in this country. So you would have to buy all Organic; which is not possible without restricting your diet even further.

You could grow all the produce yourself, or hire someone to do it for you, if you can afford to. So, the perfect diet is not practical in this country and the life styles we live in this country.

You could grow all your own food organically and drink pure water. But as soon as you are forced to send your children to school, they'll gag them with poison saturated food. But the Perfect Diet would be to grow all your food organically and drink pure water. You can grow peaches, figs, apples, grapes, Kiwi, Strawberries and all kinds of fruits to go along with your organic vegetables. Stick to drinking pure water, and you're on the Perfect Diet! But since we all know how impractical this is, we have to present an idea or ideas that are achievable for most people. So how do we come close to having the Perfect Diet, living in this country?

The obvious is just buy produce from the grocery store and wash it extra good, and make as much of that produce as you can, Organic produce. Then buy Organic 2% milk. Eat lots and lots of brown rice. Drink Lipton tea sweetened with Stevia. Buy only whole fish or fillets. No breading. Bake your own whole grain breads and don't add the sick crap to them, like vegetable oils, margarine, white flour and white granulated sugar.

Buy frozen produce when fresh is not available. Never buy canned. And use raw honey anywhere you want and as much as you want. Drink lots of pure Noni, Goji and Mangosteen juice or Goji berries. Add dried fruits and nuts to your diet. And even adding all these things beyond the ultimate Perfect Diet, you still have a near perfect diet.

Your body is 80% water. So drink 1-ounce water per 2 pounds of body weight daily to flush toxins out of your body to clean it and keep it clean inside.

And that is The Perfect Diet!

But for most of you, you will want to read on and use Chapters 6 & 7 as a guide from now on to avoid those poisons that saturate our entire food and drinks supplies. And keep the principles in mind at all times that I just discussed in the first chapters while you change to The Perfect Diet or choose to clean up your current diet by using chapters 6 and 7 as your guide.

It's not reasonable to expect everyone to get on the Perfect Diet. So that's why I am giving you the information in the next three chapters that I learned to do as I was scrambling to clean up my diet to try and add some time to my life. This information took me hundreds of hours of reading labels and researching various aspects of what I discovered.

And all that information has been filtered to exclude the things that did not help. The things that did help is what you'll be reading next. Hopefully you will use these chapters as a guide to clean up your diet, because what we know as the American diet is killing us all! Change your way of thinking and you change yourself forever!

5 -Poisons in Your Water

It is very important that I talk to you about the poisons in your water first before we get to food and drinks. The first city to provide chlorinated water in the US was Jersey City in 1908. At least 70% of the US population gets their water from systems relying on chlorine; although 90% of the water systems in the US rely on chlorination in one form or the other. Chlorine was first used in water supplies to stop typhoid. Researchers claim this actually worked, and have presented proof that chlorine kills other water borne diseases. I don't doubt any of this. As a matter of fact, if it wasn't for the chlorine in your water you would get sick shortly after drinking water in city water systems.

So I agree that the chlorine needs to be in the water to kill germs. But guess what? Chlorine kills bacteria. Oh, you already knew that! LOL But what rare few ever realize is that chlorine keeps right on being itself and kills bacteria once it's inside your body. And that is what no one is talking about. Your water supplier sure doesn't want to talk about it either.

I called our water supplier called CW&L. The Manager of CW&L certainly admitted to the chlorine and fluoride they put in our water. But he refused to agree to warn the Public about the dangers and adverse consequences of drinking and showering in their chlorinated water. I told him point blank "You need to take the fluoride out of the water. It should never have been put in our water." As he pretended to defend his position in favor of the poisons, he pointed out how beneficial fluoride is in preventing a few cavities. What he didn't want to talk about is what fluoride has to do with safe drinking water or the many cases of brittle bones, chromosome damage and other conditions known to be caused by fluoride ingestion.

The fluoride in drinking water has absolutely no benefit beyond this claim about preventing cavities. But hey, we could add Vitamin C to the water. It's good for you. Or add other things that are good for us. That is, if you don't care about clean water! Whoops! You mean CW&L has lost touch with reality and no longer realizes that our water supply is NOT the place to be adding chemicals or anything else.

Water is H2O, NOT H2O+chlorine+fluoride! I want WATER, H2O! But I can't get it. So I gotta give it to myself by getting a fluoride water filter. It would be so easy IF CW&L would stop being CWL&Dental and start being CW&L again! But they refuse. So I gotta keep using a fluoride water filter. No problem, except for the $110 to buy a fluoride water filter.

But even though chlorine and fluoride cause a host of diseases, the most significant damage that immediately affects everyone who drinks it is how chlorine kills the beneficial bacteria in your stomach and intestines. Remember, I already pointed out that chlorine is in your water to kill bacteria! Problem is,

chlorine keeps right on killing bacteria once it's inside your body! Is this good? NO. That beneficial bacteria in your stomach and intestines is required to sustain your life. As these bacteria, flora, are killed your body digests less of your food. This issue is so important that I want you to read some technical facts about this bacteria, gut flora. So I am including what Wikipedia says about this, even though most of you can just SEARCH Wikipedia for "gut flora". Here's exactly what Wikipedia states:

• **Gut flora** consists of microorganisms that live in the digestive tracts of animals and is the largest reservoir of human flora. Gut (the adjective) is synonymous with intestinal, and flora with microbiota and micro flora.

• The human body, consisting of about 100 trillion cells, carries about ten times as many microorganisms in the intestines. The metabolic activities performed by these bacteria resemble those of an organ, leading some to liken gut bacteria to a forgotten organ. It's estimated that these gut flora have around 100 times as many genes in aggregate as there are in the human genome.

• Bacteria make up most of the flora in the colon and up to 60% of the dry mass of feces. Somewhere between 300 and 1000 different species live in the gut, with most estimates at about 500. However, it is probable that 99% of the bacteria come from about 30 or 40 species. Fungi and protozoa also make up a part of the gut flora, but little is known about their activities.

• Research suggests that the relationship between gut flora and humans is not merely commensal (a non-harmful coexistence), but rather a symbiotic relationship. Though people can survive without gut flora, the microorganisms perform a host of useful functions, such as fermenting unused energy substrates, training the immune system, preventing growth of harmful, pathogenic bacteria, regulating the development of the gut, producing vitamins for the host (such as biotin and vitamin K), and producing hormones to direct the host to store fats. However, in certain conditions, some species are thought to be capable of causing disease by producing infection or increasing cancer risk for the host.

Now that you have some in depth information about the bacteria, flora, in your stomach and intestines and its tremendous importance, now I'll tell you how killing this bacteria, by drinking chlorinated water, affects you and your health. The most common condition affects how much you eat. Almost all of us drink chlorinated water our entire childhood lives. After 18 years of doing this you have significantly reduced the amount of good bacteria in your stomach and intestines. As a result, you eat a good meal, but you are hungry again within an hour and a half to two hours later. Why? Because you are mistaking the barren feeling in your stomach as hunger pains. So you eat food to feel something in your stomach.

Eating sugary foods, drinking sugary drinks and eating white flour aggravates and burns your stomach and intestines making this empty barren feeling even worse! Then heartburn begins as a further sign of this damage to your stomach and intestines. Then your intestines begin to bleed and you bleed out your bunghole, or rectum for you technically minded people. Your doctor calls this bleeding ulcers, but can't really do a thing for you; although doctors do trick people into having surgery to correct this. But is there any condition that doctors do NOT claim you need surgery for?!? Yes you need surgery so doctors can make big bucks off your disease and suffering.

But for you to be cured of bleeding ulcers, you're gonna need to learn what I am telling you. I wish I could charge a small percentage of the huge amounts of money the information in this book saves you. Then compare that to what the medical industry charges you to treat and drug your diseases and medical conditions but never cure you. Natural healing is the only way you can be cured and costs a fraction of what doctors charge without ever curing you.

What can I do to replenish this good bacteria killed by chlorine? There are several things you can do. You can take probiotics. That's what I did. Believe me. I didn't know much of anything when I was learning the things I talk about in this book. So I used myself as a guinea pig to experiment and test these things to save my own life, or end up on dialysis by 2008 or dead by 2009 as the doctors insisted. I started taking probiotics. I started out just taking some Lactobacillus acidophilus and B. Lactis, also known as Acidophilus complex. Once I started taking Dr. Ohirra's Probiotics 12 Plus I started noticing that I wasn't hungry shortly after eating and my stomach felt much better.

I am still taking Dr. Ohirra's Probiotics from time to time and take the Acidophilus complex daily, usually more than once a day with meals. Buy the Acidophilus with the most active cultures. I use the one with 1 billion live organisms per capsule. Capsules are much easier to digest and therefore provide the greatest benefit compared to caplets or tablets. Acidophilus is the easiest pro-biotic to find. It's one of two bacteria found in yogurt. Probiotics with 10-12 different bacteria or more are a little harder to find, but provide the greatest health benefits; especially a natural probiotics product such as Dr. Ohhira's Probiotics.

Eating fresh, raw fruits and vegetables aid in the production of beneficial bacteria in your stomach and intestines too. The enzymes in raw fruits and vegetables are the key to this aid, and do so many other beneficial things to improve your health and heal your body. So eat as much fresh, raw fruits and vegetables as you can. There are lots of books explaining the endless health benefits of fresh fruits and vegetables, so I will not go into this in depth. Fresh fruits and vegetables provide generous amounts of fiber to protect your stomach and intestines, aid in digestion, nourish and heal damaged cells and promote regular bowel movements.

People whose diets are lacking in fresh fruits and vegetables and fiber rarely have bowel movements every day. Fact is, you should have a bowel movement not too long after each meal. Most of you will say that's crazy. No one has a bowel movement after each meal or most meals! But what I say to you is this... it's NOT crazy either. Want some proof?

Oki dokey people! Any of you ever have children? Ah ha! You only changing poopy diapers ONCE each day! I think NOT! When you are born and a baby, your stomach and intestines are healthy. You know, before you start killing your insides with chlorinated water, antibiotics, sugars and more. So you poop after each meal usually. But as you bombard your intestines with all these poisons, your body goes to work trying to protect itself against all these poisons. As a result, your intestines get coated with mucus.

Mucus looks like snot and boogers mixed together; which you see in your poop quite often. Once this mucus coats your intestines, your intestines have a harder and harder time of digesting and absorbing nutrients. In addition, you start developing pockets in your intestines which your poop begins to move into. You can have as much as 5-10 pounds of poop stuck in these pockets in your intestines; which stay in your intestines rotting for years, causing even more discomfort and health problems.

Doing a colon cleanse will do a lot in solving this problem. There are lots of different colon cleanses on the market. Most of them aren't very good. But I have tried a few of them. The best ones I have found are called Colonix and Almighty Cleanse. But here's a link you can go to and read about the top colon cleansers and make your own choice. www.detoxreviews.com If you do any internal cleanses, make sure you do a colon cleanse first. That way, if you did a liver cleanse, kidney cleanse or any other internal cleanse you won't cause yourself problems by overloading your intestines with poisons. So cleanse your colon, then do other cleanses to be safe and as effective as possible.

Although the cause of Elvis Presley's death was ruled as a heart attack, his doctors had treated Elvis for chronic constipation for over a decade before his death, and now believe Elvis's death was actually caused by chronic constipation. Elvis' autopsy revealed that Elvis' digestive system was a real mess when he died and that Elvis would've have lived longer if he had a colostomy. I know that doing a colon cleanse certainly helped me. The proof was how it made me feel better and lighter inside and by looking at my own poop when I was doing colon cleanses. I go by results, not the price of the product or the sales pitch and advertisements about the product.

I want to point out to you right now that it was necessary for me to talk about the poisons in your water first, before I talked about anything else for a very good reason. As you read this book there are many things I recommend that you put into your body. But these vitamins, herbs, foods and other items have to be digested properly. So the more beneficial bacteria you have in your stomach and intestines, the better you digest these items and thus, the more you benefit from taking them.

In some people these vitamins, herbs and foods may seem to do you very little good if the beneficial bacteria in your stomach and intestines is greatly depleted. So, for these vitamins, herbs and foods to do you more good and benefit you more greatly you will need to take probiotics as the first thing to do. Then you will get the greatest benefits from taking supplements, herbs and healthy foods in the most cost effective and efficient manner.

About the most important thing you can do about the poisons in your water is to get some type of water filter. You need one for your drinking and cooking water and one for your shower. Yes, you need a shower filter. But first let's look at the solution for needing a water filter. You can buy inexpensive faucet end carbon water filters. Years ago, we bought a Water Pik faucet end filter. It does a lot of good for about $20.

You can buy easily replaceable carbon filter cartridges for about $5 each or a 4 pack for around $16. We got ours at Lowe's back in the 80's and used it till we got a cylinder shaped counter top carbon water filter from HSN. These filters are worth the money if that is all you can afford or care to invest at first. What you really need is a fluoride filter. A carbon filter only filters out about 90% of the chlorine, some dirt and other impurities, but not a speck of fluoride. Fluoride is a smaller particle and requires a better filter to eliminate it.

Fluoride filters – Fluoride filters are my filter of choice. Sure, I'd like to have a whole house osmosis filtration system, but the fluoride water filter we use is really great. The chlorine and fluoride give tap water a bitter taste which you get use to after drinking it that way for years. But I always do a little test to show people the difference between water and chlorinated, fluoridated water.

I take two identical glasses. Pour chlorinated, fluoridated water in one glass and pure water from our fluoride water filter in the other glass, and ask them to tell me if they can tell any difference and which one they like the best. 100% of the people so far always say the water that came from the fluoride water filter is the best and know which is which. I also ask them "What does the water from the fluoride filter taste like?" Their answer "Nothing" or "It doesn't have any taste". I tell them "Right, because it's WATER!"

When we first got our fluoride water filter, my wife and I would giggle every time after drinking some water. Hey, don't bash us! hehe We couldn't help it. Every drink of water going down our throats is pure and tasteless! Neither of us had ever had that experience. We felt highly privileged to be drinking water so pure. We even thought it was stupid that we felt that way about a water filter! Problem is, we are worse about it now than we were at the first. I love that pure water. You can drink all you want and it does absolutely no harm, and does so much good for your body and your health.

Having pure water from our fluoride water filter may have been the #1 factor in saving my life or at least sparing my life for years so far. Even doctors will tell you that your kidneys love water. And the fact that I was diagnosed with chronic kidney disease a few months earlier made pure water become the thing I began to consume the most. **You need one ounce of water for every two pounds of body weight daily.** For me that's around three quarts daily.

I never drank that much water in my life, and the older I got the less water I drank. Fortunately for me, the past 30 years I've been drinking filtered water. I sometimes think about how much chlorine I have NOT consumed and the internal damage that comes with drinking tap water. Your body has to filter out every bit of that chlorine and fluoride, and almost all of that work is handled by your kidneys. Once your kidneys get saturated with so much poison that they can't remove all of it from your body as quickly as you pour and stuff those poisons down your throat, your kidneys will begin to fail. I'll tell you how that happened to me in Chapter 12.

What about a shower filter? I believe a shower filter is at least as important as having a filter on your drinking and cooking water. I never thought about having a shower filter my whole life and honestly had never heard of such a thing. I didn't know anything about shower filters until after I bought one. Now, sometimes I get to thinking a shower filter is more important than a filter for drinking and cooking water; which bolsters my opinion that you need both and should see them both as necessities. The main reason I believe this is because **you soak up about ten times as much chlorine and fluoride in the shower as you generally do through drinking and cooking water.**

Water causes the pores in your skin to expand; which allows greater absorption into your body and bloodstream. After we got our shower filter I could tell right off that the water coming out of the shower filter no longer had that chemical chlorine smell. I even got a large glass of tap water to sniff in the shower; which I then sniffed the water coming out of the shower filter. The tap water had that familiar chlorine smell, and the filtered shower water had no smell. Then I just left it to hopefully do what I bought it for.

A few weeks later my wife and I both got a good surprise. We have had burning itchy places on our bodies over the years. We blamed cold weather, taking too many showers and maybe a few other things, but never got rid of those itchy red places. When I looked back soon after this, I realized while in the shower that those red itchy places were the exact places where the most shower water hits my body.

Our good surprise was that we no longer had those red itchy places just 3 weeks after installing our shower filter! I got on the INTERNET to SEARCH for something to explain our good surprise. As it turns out, the chlorine in tap water destroys the oils in your skin and... and... YOUR HAIR! Got dandruff! I bet you do after burn drying your scalp with chlorinated water! I repeat... the chlorine in your shower water dries out your skin, scalp and hair by destroying the oils in your skin, scalp and hair!

Don't calm down yet! LOL Here's what could be the worst part... (I say this very sincerely and make the following comparison to save lives, and for this reason, the following should not offend anyone.) We all know Hitler used chlorine gas to murder millions of people. So, there's not a one of us who does not know how wrong this is, and should not be done to anyone. But guess what? Almost every one of you are doing the same thing to yourself, and doing it daily in most cases.

You got that hot chlorinated water steaming up the shower enclosure and that chlorinated steam goes right into your lungs and into your blood stream as fast as possible. Remember when I pointed out that YOU are the one who made YOU sick? Who told you chlorine gas was safe! Oh yeah...I forgot to mention that HUGE fact that the result of ingesting chlorine damages every cell it comes in contact with. Search the INTERNET to find information about all the various specific damage chlorine is known to do to your body.

Where do I buy probiotics, a carbon or fluoride water filter and a shower filter? I confess to buying them all off Ebay. You can also get some probiotics from Puritans Pride – www.puritans.com. And of course, there are lots of places on the INTERNET. We have bought from Puritan's Pride for almost 30 years. We were buying from Nutrition Headquarters who were later bought by Puritan's Pride. We buy vitamins, herbs, soap and other items from Puritans Pride too. We place an order every 2 or 3 months.

The shower filter we use is made by Crystal Quest. Search Ebay for KDF shower filter. Shower filters use a special carbon filter known as a KDF filter. This type shower filter uses a carbon filter which is designed for filtering hot water. If you run hot water through any carbon filter that is not specified as a KDF filter, the hot water will cause your carbon filter to dissolve. So make sure you purchase a KDF filter and don't be running hot water through any of the carbon or fluoride filters you use for your drinking and cooking water; which is connected to your kitchen faucet.

Beware that when we bought our first shower filter in early 2007, we couldn't find one at any store in this hub of commerce City of 70,000 people. Hard to believe, but it's true. And of course, SEARCH the INTERNET for the store of your choice if you don't care for Ebay.

As for a water filter for cooking and drinking water, I always recommend a disposable counter-top fluoride filter from Pure Water Essentials. The one we use is: http://purewateressentials.com/ct00130.html.

It costs $100 plus shipping of around ten dollars. It lasts for years. Pure

Water Essentials sells all types of water filters. So you can browse their site and find what's best for you. But I have recommended this filter to everyone so far.

What about bottled water? The simple answer is...don't be a fool! Buying bottled water is foolish and a waste of money, unless there are some odd circumstances I haven't thought of. If the gas company has fracked your water supply you could need bottled water. Fracked water will ruin your water filter in no time! Bottled water contains more than water. I looked and looked and looked for bottled WATER, but could only find bottled water with several other ingredients! The best bottled water I found was Ozarka. It has the fewest ingredients. You can get about ONE THOUSAND times as much filtered water by buying a counter top water filter than you get buying bottled water.

Some bottled water is just tap water in a bottle too. And your fluoride filtered water is pure. Bottled water never is. So your body has to filter out those added ingredients. I bought bottled water one time, and that was enough to convince me to never buy any more.

Remember, the information in this book is not only to prevent and cure disease, it can and will save you lots and lots of money. And that's the bottom line 'cause...whoops, don't want Stone Cold Steve Austin claiming I was using his catch phrase. So that's the bottom line 'cause...if I told you otherwise, I'd be lying.

You need to remember that I am extremely happy to still be alive. So that deep joy is ingrained into what I tell you in this book. I am so happy to know all of this. So happy that all of it is true proven science. And I'm so happy to be sharing it with you. I thought doctors cured people, until I went to them for a cure in 2006 and didn't get cured of anything.

So change your attitude by knowing there is a cure for all disease. Raise the pH of your body so disease can not exist. Drink as pure a water as possible and use a shower filter. And correct the 3 main diet deficiencies – Vitamin C, Omega-3 and Magnesium.

That's a great start. Now that we've purified all your water, let's see how we can avoid poisons in our drinks.

6 -Poisons in Your Drinks

Now here's the subject that almost killed me and still shocks me and pisses me off sometimes - the poisons in our drinks. I have been an organic gardener since 1981, so I have eaten very healthy food all these years. I even trimmed the fat off all the meat I ate, to be safe. Sure I ate some bad foods. But it wasn't very often or very much. And even though I was the healthiest eater among family, friends and acquaintances, quite often people would say "Watch what you eat". "Oh I do" I would tell them, and it was the truth. I only had one cold/flu since 1981 and no serious illness for nearly two decades, so my health confirmed I was eating right. And guess what? I really was!

But you know what no one EVER told me? What I never told myself either? No one ever said "Watch what you DRINK". Oh how I wish with all my mind and body that someone would've told me that! Oh how I wish I had told myself that! But no one did, and I never did. I didn't tell anyone to watch what they drink either. But I was good at telling people "watch what you eat".

I know most of you are wondering what in the blues blazes am I talking about! Don't feel bad about it. I felt like Columbus setting sail to sail off the edge of the earth and like Lewis and Clark westward explorations. I was heading into unknown territory! Why the very idea of thinking something bad about beloved companies who make Coke, Pepsi, Dr. Pepper, Ocean Spray, Gatorade, Welch's and the rest.

All their products are verified "safe" by the FDA. But what their products had done to my health compelled and convinced me to at least consider bad things about those products. At first I was lost as to figure out what blew out my kidneys. I tell the story in Chapter 12 about how I came to learn almost all the cures I have proven and learned about. I also tell what happened that forced me to face up to reality as it really is, about everything I was eating, drinking or coming into contact with.

When I began to learn the magnitude of how poisoned our drinks supply is, my incurable chronic kidney disease began to improve; instead of getting progressively worse and ending in death. The only options doctors gave me was dialysis within 2 years and death likely shortly thereafter. I would need a kidney transplant at that point to avoid death. So I was determined to find out what caused my kidneys to fail, even though the doctors could never tell me. It was hypertension that blew my kidneys, but they couldn't tell me what caused my high blood pressure either. One doctor said it was probably salt. But none of my metabolic tests ever backed that up or even hinted to such a thing. So all I could do is wonder what caused this. I was lost as anyone could be and felt so helpless. But one day that all began to change.

As I began to pay attention to how I felt; examining, scrutinizing and analyzing how I felt all day long, I began to recognize a reoccurring bad sick feeling. I had been scrambling to find something to drink to replace the sugar soaked sweet tea I loved to guzzle down at every meal. So I got some fruit juices that said they were made from concentrate. Gee. I'm about to drink some totally healthy fruit juice and not only that, it's concentrated fruit juice! Yippee. Roll out the success mat. I've got something healthy to drink, and lots of it. But then, here comes that mean a-hole, Mr. Reality and Mr. Facts to boot, and there goes my fruit juices! The problem is that I thought concentrate meant they boiled the fruit juice down to make a concentrated form of that juice.

I was wrong. The FDA guidelines for claiming something as concentrate basically means packed with as much sugar or high fructose corn syrup as they choose to put in their products. I kept reading fruit juice cans and jars looking for any juice that was not made from concentrate. As I read the labels I keep noticing high fructose corn syrup in the ingredients. My wife and I kept throwing our hands up in disbelief about this. The reality is, that **once you start trying to eliminate high fructose corn syrup, the grocery store becomes a much smaller place.**

When I started looking for fruit juices without high fructose corn syrup, I was still chugging' down the cranberry juice. I was just blind to the facts. I had been drinking this most popular brand of cranberry juice and bragged about how healthy it was for me. Of course, I hadn't read the label either. Turns out it has more sugar declared on the label than your most popular brands of soda pops. I thought, no this can't be true. Something as good for you as cranberry juice and they packed it with poison. It made no sense. It couldn't be true. OR maybe I was just full of you know what. It rhymes with mit.

I drank some cranberry juice and within 10 minutes I had that tense sick feeling again. I realized that I had that feeling every time I drank some cranberry juice after my kidneys failed. But it was so out of place and downright insane that something so good for you was really extremely bad for you. I had been drinking almost a quart every day for almost 3 years. All that time I thought I was so smart to be drinking cranberry juice almost every day. I never even stopped to think it might be bad for you. I tossed out the last of the cranberry juice and kept on looking for anything without high fructose corn syrup. Your liver turns excess sugar into LDL, bad cholesterol, causing high blood pressure.

Boy, what a bummer! I was down to water and milk. And at that time, I hadn't gotten my fluoride water filter I talked about in the previous chapter. At that point I was starting to make it a habit to read every label. So **I was wondering what poisons I was gonna find in my milk** and leave me with nothing but water to drink. I tried switching to 2% milk. But it tasted weak to me. While I went back and forth between whole milk and 2% milk, I researched the information about the various types of milk. Whole milk is at least 3.25% milk fat. 2% milk is 2% milk fat. And skim and non-fat milk contain no more than

0.5% milk fat by weight. The significance of the fat content is that the growth hormones, antibiotics and other chemicals are concentrated and stored in fat cells in mammals; which includes cattle and humans. So the more fat in the milk, the more of these drugs and chemicals you will be consuming.

When you try and switch from whole milk to a lower fat milk, you will probably have a hard time and want to give up. Hey, I hope you switch overnight! But most can't do that. What I found out is that your body and mind are addicted to the chemicals you taste in whole milk. You think you like that momentary pleasure. So you have to deal with what's going on in your mind. This is true about any and every food you are addicted to. If you crave it or make excuses for not switching to a healthier version of a product, then you are addicted to that product. I hear that about milk only second to soda pops.

Attitude and proper mind set – I want you to know that as I write this book, I have to keep trying to get the point across to you that since we all naively believe our food, drinks and water supplies are really safe, I have to work hard to get it across to you how absolutely false that is. In reality, rare few food products we ingest are safe. The FDA declares products safe as long as they don't kill you quickly. So stop agreeing to consume what kills you a little bit later than if you had taken cyanide pills.

It took about 5 years of regular use of a quart of cranberry juice, 20 oz. Gatorade, 3 sodas and a quart of sweet tea a day to cause my kidney failure. And I never saw it coming. Why would I? I was eating extremely healthy and drinking Gatorade to get my electrolytes and cranberry juice full of anti-oxidants and cancer preventing Lipton sweet tea.

Don't be scared. Be informed!

If I skipped all these parts about attitude and mind set, you would most likely miss the boat on actually curing yourself or preventing the diseases you will get by trusting the food companies and medical professionals. You need to have a chip on your shoulder at the grocery store that pushes you to read labels in the store and never bring the poisons home in the first place. **Everything you buy is poisoned. All you can do is limit the amount of poisons you purchase and ingest.** And when you ingest poisons in liquid form, your body digests and absorbs a far greater amount of these poisons.

What about soda pops? Sorry, it's all bad news when it comes to soda pops. The acidity of all sodas is roughly 3.0. Problem is, that your body's pH needs to be between 6.0 and 7.3. The further below 7.3 you get, the more your pH adversely affects and impedes body metabolisms. In simple words, drinking sodas makes your body ripe for disease just because of the extreme acidity. The HMF in high fructose corn syrup, hydroxymethylfurfural, has been linked to DNA damage in humans. HMF content rises as high fructose corn syrup gets warm. Once it reaches 120 degrees Fahrenheit, HMF levels rise dramatically.

Then add to that the sodium benzoate that has been proven to have the ability to switch off vital parts of DNA in a cell's mitochondria. And when you add Vitamin C in with the sodium benzoate it causes benzene, a known carcinogenic substance. The mitochondria is called the power station of the DNA. So this damage is severe and leads to serious cell malfunction. This damage is linked to such diseases as Parkinson's disease, many neuro-degenerative diseases and most of all the whole aging process.

Now what I am about to add about sodas is my opinion from my experiences with sodas, what I have researched and what I concluded on my own. I don't have any proof beyond my opinion and experiences. So you can choose whether to believe the following. I concluded that high fructose corn syrup mutates your genes. High fructose corn syrup is made with genetically altered corn in a 3 step process using genetically altered enzymes.

The manufacturers of this poison won't tell you exactly how it's made and advertise what seems to be a white lie recipe for high fructose corn syrup. It shouldn't surprise anyone. They have never admitted the scientific facts about the poisons in their HFCS. They have even started calling HFCS "corn sugar" to try and hide HFCS as an ingredient in products. But it may very well be the DNA altering actions of the ingredients in sodas that I have concluded to be gene-mutating actions. I will continue being open to the facts in order to reach a final decision about this.

What is bad about sodas? DNA altering HMF, DNA altering sodium benzoate, a 3.0 acidity and possible gene-mutating high fructose corn syrup; which is also where the HMF comes from. And you get that wonderful sugar burn with every drink, and the acid also eats away at your teeth and gums. It sure didn't take any more for me to stop drinking sodas. I went from drinking at least one thousand sodas a year to somewhere around 10 to 12 sodas a year. As I look back at this, I have no doubt as to why my kidneys failed.

All these serious poisons, not to mention the fact that one 12-ounce soda pop shuts down your immune system for about 6 hours. Technically it does not shut your immune system down. It's just that your immune system is pre-occupied with trying to remove all the ingredients in that soda that your body can't use. That is all it can do for about six hours. Drink a soda every 6 hours and you in essence have no immune system working to heal you. How do you have a chance against sickness in this condition!

So what about tea? Tea is really good for you. I still drink tea and have all along. We switched to Lipton decaffeinated tea, but still couldn't stand swigging down all that sugar for sweetened tea. We used less and less sugar to see if that would work. You're supposed to use 4 cups per gallon. But we only used half that amount for years. So we started using less and less. It was OK in moderation, but I wasn't liking it very well after all those years of real sugary tea.

One day we heard about an herbal sweetener called Stevia. Stevia is 30 times as sweet as sugar. We used less than a teaspoon in a gallon of tea. At first I kept saying "This tea just isn't sweet at all" and started to abandon Stevia altogether. I decided that before I did that I would do a little test. So I made a gallon pitcher of tea.

I poured a few ounces into a glass, unsweetened. Then I added the Stevia to the pitcher of tea. Drank one, then the other. Ah ha! Now I could tell the Stevia really was making the tea sweet. The problem was that the tea wasn't giving my mouth that sugar burn that gives you cotton mouth, dry mouth. I then realized that I had been addicted to that sugar burn, and had been swigging down tea to get that sugar burn sensation. It's the same kind of mind addiction that all those chemicals in whole milk give you. As long as you remember that sugar burn is the proof of how bad sugar is, you will make the switch to Stevia. I'll cover this some more in the chapter – Poisons in Your Food, when I discuss sweeteners.

Solutions and Chapter Summary – I'm sorry to sink the Titanic about all your favorite drinks like sodas and fruit juices. But really, basically all the drink products on the market are flavored sugar waters. And most of them are packed with the worst poison of all in my experiences, research and opinion... high fructose corn syrup. You need to assume every drink product is packed with high fructose corn syrup, and check the labels to see IF you can find something that does not have HFCS.

When it comes to juices, look for products that say "NOT FROM CONCENTRATE". These words will be in plain sight. But even when the product says "NOT FROM CONCENTRATE", you still need to read the labels and see what the ingredients are. If it has high fructose corn syrup, don't buy it. The only juices we buy are Simply Orange, Florida Nature and Tropicana orange juices and Musselman's apple juice. The Tropicana orange juice in our refrigerator right now says "NEVER FROM CONCENTRATE" on the front of the cartoon. Always read the ingredients list to make sure it doesn't contain HFCS.

And even the juices that say NOT FROM CONCENTRATE still aren't very good for you. Most orange juice makers grind the entire orange, then store that in underground tanks and let it sit for months before sending it to the stores for us to buy.

That's my findings for juices that are worth buying if you care anything about your health. I told you already how tiny the grocery store gets once you start reading labels to eliminate high fructose corn syrup from your diet! This is one of the main reasons I wrote this book. You can try hundreds of different juices, read hundreds of juice labels and only about 2% of the juice products available are healthy and actually safe to drink.

In addition to Simply Orange, Florida Nature and Tropicana orange juices and Musselman's apple juice, you can drink 2% or skim milk, Unsweetened or

Stevia sweetened tea and filtered water. One juice I failed to mention was tomato juice. Tomato juice is pretty good for you. The only drawback is if you absolutely have to avoid salt, you shouldn't drink tomato juice. Tomato juice is packed heavily with salt. Tomato juice contains about 650mg of sodium per 8 ounce serving; which translates to roughly 5000mg of salt per 48 ounce can.

If you're going to drink milk, then simply drink 2% milk. If you can find it and afford it, buy Organic 2% milk. I think even Organic Whole milk would have less poisons in it than non-organic 2% milk. I drink Organic 2% milk when they have it at Kroger's. That stuff Wal-Mart sells has a slightly funky taste. That makes it suspicious to me. So I buy Organic milk only from Kroger. It's $2 a gallon more than regular milk, but well worth it. Use less milk so you buy less often. Organic milk keeps fresh weeks after regular milks have soured too.

I just recently tried that new soda pop called Sierra Mist Natural. It's a lemon lime soda that, believe it or not, does not contain high fructose corn syrup or man-made artificial sweeteners. It just contains sugar. The ingredients are carbonated water, sugar, citric acid, natural flavor and Potassium citrate. Citric acid is organic. Potassium citrate is a Potassium salt of citric acid. Sugar is a processed food substance and carbonated water is water that has had carbon dioxide gas under pressure dissolved in it. So that's a pretty good soda, except for the acidic carbonated water and the empty calories of the sugar.

But it doesn't have a yucky chemical taste to it compared to sodas with high fructose corn syrup and sodium benzoate. That's a tremendous improvement over all other sodas. So I'll be drinking a few of them. I'll be splitting them with my wife since I only drink half a can at a time now.

Sometimes Coke and Dr. Pepper put out a limited supply of their products that substitute pure cane sugar for high fructose corn syrup. I haven't ever been able to get any. But, it's your chance to have a soda pop without that sick high fructose corn syrup or pukey aspartame or some other man made artificial chemical sweetener.

You need to take it seriously when it comes to what you drink. There are only a rare few products that aren't all bad for you. Our drinks are more saturated with poisons than our food supplies. The information in this chapter can guide you away from the worst products.

There is lots and lots of information on diet and eating right. But rarely does any of that information include avoiding poisons in your foods. That is what I am going to talk to you about now.....Poisons in Your Food. And a some of that is about Poisons that ARE your food, like white flour and white sugar.

7 -Poisons in Your Food

What do I mean by poisons in your food? I mean the chemicals that are added to food products. The most well-known are preservatives, dyes and additives of all sorts. I'm also talking about white flour, white granulated sugar, high fructose corn syrup, vegetable oils and red meat. I sometimes refer to these as poison foods. There are so many chemicals in our food supply. Quite a few of them are not necessary and are put in food products to addict you to those products. Yes, you heard me correctly.

Food companies intentionally put chemicals in your food to addict you to their products. Of course, food companies won't admit this or even talk about it. But they also never talk about any proof that their chemicals are safe. Why act like it's some secret that food companies want you to buy as much of their products as they can get you to. I've never seen any indication that they have any morals or care about you and your health one bit. All they care about is greater sales and profits to please their stockholders and their lust for money, greed. All they have to do is get FDA approval for their poisons and poison saturated products and it's all legal, approved and FDA certified safe.

As long as you don't get sick or drop dead immediately after eating their products, the FDA claims it's "safe". You are not a person or human being to corporations. You are a consumer who has what they want...your money. Has one corporation been there at the bedside of any of the millions of people their products have killed? I think NOT!

The best advice I can give anyone to inspire them to get serious about avoiding the saturation of poisons in your food is this – **Always have a chip on your shoulder when you're at the grocery store.** And no I don't mean be an a-hole to people or tackle those who look at you wrong! LOL I mean **read food labels and refuse to buy the hordes of harmful poisonous products.** I can promise you that you will begin to get furious once you start reading the labels on products after you learn about the poisons in those products.

You also need to learn what those labels mean and not be fooled by the massive trickery food companies use to trick you into buying their products. It takes more time at the grocery store, but your life is on the line and so is your health. Start right now and read all the labels on the products you already have in your home. This is exactly what my wife and I did when I blew out my kidneys in 2006. Make reading labels a habit in your life.

I thought I knew the difference between healthy and harmful foods until I started reading ALL the labels. And that was a major factor in saving my life. I'll tell you more about this later on. But for now, let's continue about food labels, what they really mean and some of the things to look for as you work to keep these poisons out of your homes and out of your bodies. Reading labels and knowing what they mean is the most important thing to learn about finding the poisons in your food and drinks so you can avoid them.

Here's what the FDA says about the ingredient labels on products:

All the ingredients, listed in order of predominance by weight. In other words, the ingredient that weighs the most is listed first, and the ingredient that weighs the least is last.

So the first ingredient could be as much as 99% of the product. And the second ingredient could be as much as 49% of the product by weight. These are the extremes possible in any product. If a product lists any of the toxic poisons mentioned in this book in the first three ingredients, that product should be on your hit list as a product to eliminate or greatly limit and restrict its use. If the poison is toward the middle of the label, consider it a moderate health risk. If the poison is listed toward the end, consider it a mild risk if used regularly.

Reading labels MUST become a way of life. Even after years of reading labels we still make mistakes and buy products in every category; high risk, moderate and mild. IF I had it my way, food companies would be required to put labels on poison soaked products that say "Regular use of this product will cause diseases and eventually kill you." But hey, that would be honest. So that's NOT going to happen.

Take high fructose corn syrup for example: This DNA altering poison is in everything, and I mean everything. The most harmful products that contain high fructose corn syrup are fruit juices and soda pops. And yes, I said fruit juices. I don't know of any more harmful products than fruit juices and soda pops. They are not only saturated with poisons, as a liquid they are far more easily digested than any solid foods and therefore far more harmful. I went into some of the specific details about these drinks in the "Poisons in Your Drinks" chapter.

Now I will tackle some real problems with popular food items and tell you why you should avoid them and what you can do about substituting healthier products for those poisonous food products. Let's get started!

What about bread? Whole wheat or white? Well, the easy way is just to say eat whole wheat breads and flour. But most people don't know why they should choose whole wheat, and a lot of us can't even buy whole wheat buns, cakes, cookies, etc. You certainly can't find a restaurant that serves whole wheat bread, buns or rolls. Yes it's insane. But that's the reality we are forced to deal with. I have never understood why whole wheat bread is sometimes hard to find and nearly impossible to get in restaurants. You need to tell every restaurant you do business with that you want whole wheat bread, buns, cakes and cookies, and that you will take your business elsewhere if they don't start providing it. I doubt it will do much good, even though it's the right thing to do.

Restaurants are food companies too. So they had rather sell you white bread and vegetable oil soaked food than to take the time to care about the health and welfare of its customers. I don't believe restaurants care what customers want. At least I don't have any proof that they do. If you can find a restaurant that serves whole wheat bread or fries their foods in Canola oil, then you've found a restaurant that at least cares a little about your health.

Now, what to buy at the grocery stores – If you're at the grocery store and see loaves of bread that claim they're whole wheat, look again. Look at the label. Most of what is called whole wheat is not. Food companies label it whole wheat, but when you read the label you see the first ingredient is "enriched wheat flour". Sounds good, right? WRONG!

What enriched wheat flour really is, is white flour with vitamins. What you have to look for is breads that list the first ingredient as "whole wheat flour" or "stone ground whole wheat flour". Otherwise it's only gonna be white flour in that bread. Tricky, misleading labeling is just one of the ways food corporations retain the level of poisons in food products while tricking you into believing their products are not only safe, but healthy and good for you. Nonsense!

Did you know that white flour is a drug? There is no such thing as a white flour plant. So where does white flour come from? It comes from wheat. Food companies take wheat and remove everything from the wheat that has real nutritional value and you get white flour. They remove the wheat bran and the wheat germ and end up with that drug called white flour. You can buy white flour real cheap.

Wheat bran and wheat germ are expensive and usually have to be bought from so-called health food stores; even though you can sometimes buy wheat bran and wheat germ at your grocery store. It's shocking to learn how food companies strip wheat of all its nutritional value and sell what's left, white flour. White flour eventually causes diarrhea and intestinal bleeding. This is caused by lack of fiber, and of course, if you've ever taken a slice of white bread and smashed it into as small a ball as you can, then you have already seen the proof of how white flour has no fiber. You eat the white bread and then scramble to get more fiber in your diet; when all you have to do is eat whole wheat bread and make sure it's really whole wheat. Then you would have plenty of fiber.

Trying to avoid white flour can become a real pain in the ass because of how limited the supply of real whole wheat bread is, and because of how food companies tend to rely on that drug called white flour to addict you to their products. You buy a greasy burger at a fast food restaurant and it comes on white bread so it doesn't interfere with the taste of the grease soaked burger. Whole wheat has some nutritional value, so it also has some taste to it. You want a whole wheat cake, but can never find a whole wheat cake mix. You want whole wheat cookies, but nobody sells them. You want whole wheat buns, but you can hardly ever find them either.

So what's a person to do? You can always get a bread maker for about $70-100 and make your own. Or you can substitute whole wheat flour for white flour in recipes. You can also add some whole grains like crushed flax seed or whole wheat flour to the recipe. Adding wheat bran and wheat germ to recipes also brings some nutritional value to recipes. One thing we do is use half whole wheat flour in raisin bread. You're supposed to use bread flour. But you can use whole wheat flour as long as you add a teaspoon of wheat gluten for each cup of whole grain flour.

So when it comes to buying bread, remember to read the labels and only buy bread whose first ingredient is whole wheat flour or Stone ground whole wheat. And do not be fooled by the hordes of breads that say whole wheat on the package, but the first ingredient is white flour with vitamins; known as enriched wheat flour. There are also other whole grain breads besides wheat, like rye and multi-grain breads. When I eat out, it's at Subway's 9 times out of 10. And I always get multi-grain bread for every sandwich; not to mention the pile of chopped fresh veggies on every sandwich.

If I haven't made it clear, do not eat white bread. That means no white bread, hot dog buns, hamburger buns, dinner rolls, crescent rolls, cakes, cobblers, donuts, pastries and on and on and on. Look for whole wheat versions of all of these food items or do without them, or at least eat them in moderation. But don't make a habit of doing so. It's not worth the damage to your health; especially when you could be eating wholesome whole grain products with the fiber and nutrients your body needs. You'll feel a lot better about yourself and enjoy a much healthier body the more you choose healthy foods, and the less you choose the unhealthy foods that the grocery store shelves are packed with.

Sure you gotta spend time to learn and do all of this! But isn't your life worth the effort? Is your health worth the effort? Isn't your financial health worth it? And aren't the lives of your family and loved ones and their health and well-being worth the effort?

Making these changes in diet and lifestyle certainly is hard at first, mainly because you are so set in your ways. It's up to you to do the right thing for you and your families. I know you can do this. And the more you learn and put into practice, the more positive results you get, the more you want to learn and get to doing this. And you WILL get those results as long as you make the effort.

Meat, meat and more meat – What meat should I eat? The best answer is none, you shouldn't eat meat at all. I'll go into detail about red meat in just a few minutes. But for now, let's learn something about meat in general. Meat is dead animal flesh. We fatten animals on corporate farms, feeding and injecting these animal with all kinds of drugs and chemicals, kill them systematically, skin them and cut their dead flesh into pieces and parts; which is what you buy at the grocery store.

We make up all kinds of names for these dead animal parts and flesh to try and fool ourselves into thinking we are eating something good and healthy. Millions of Americans even take dead animal parts and smoke them on their charcoal grills; saturating them with smoke and soot that tastes good, but is poison to your body. We eat the dead flesh of cows, pigs, turkeys and chickens. Quite a few people eat deer, elk, bison and an array of other dead animal flesh and parts.

Don't get me wrong. IF you can get any meat that comes from outside the corporate food companies, that meat has avoided the saturation of chemicals that are in all meat sold by corporations. You can't chase a deer down and make him drink soda pops or fruit juice to poison the deer meat. You can't inject wild deer with antibiotics and growth hormones either. The only chance of wild animals having poisons in their systems is if they have been drinking or eating chemicals that come from the massive pollution of our air, water and land by corporations.

But humans are not supposed to be meat eaters. We don't have the teeth to be meat eaters. Meat eaters have some spiked teeth so they can rip and shred meat. Humans do not. Human teeth are for chewing vegetation and fish. But no one ever talks about this, no matter how many so-called health books you read. No, we just can't bear to be honest about things. The truth might offend someone, or cut back on the sales of their book or other things. I wouldn't even begin writing this book for a few years because of that fact.

I have been attacked, slandered, hated, threatened and even had a guy pull a gun on me in Public for stating some of these facts. I have been warned by dozens of people that I am going to get someone killed by telling them how to cure themselves of diseases. All of this is insane and complete nonsense on their part. How flax seed oil, Fish oil or vitamins could kill someone is unfounded and unheard of! But quite honestly, a lot of these lunatics are in the medical profession and/or their christianity has taught them to ignore God's natural cures in favor of the sorcery and quackery the medical profession invented over the past 75 years. Even if there is no GOD, man has been using cures from nature since man first existed.

Telling anyone anything besides go to the doctor is what they pretend is me trying to get people killed. Problem with that nonsense is that I have never told anyone NOT to go to the doctor. I only tell people that IF they want to be cured, going to the doctor is not the thing to do, since doctors have no cures. If you lose your car keys, do you look on the TV and not find them and give up and never drive your car again! No you don't. You keep looking until you find them!

And people want to accuse ME of trying to get people killed for telling you to do the same thing when it comes to your health and life! Keep going to your sorcerers disguised as doctors WHILE you cure yourself. **Having a doctor to send blood tests to the lab will help you realize that you really are curing**

yourself, preventing disease or at the least, getting better. But I'll have more to say about this later on. For now, let's get back to Poisons in our Food.

The American diet – Dead cow flesh – Everyone is on that savage diet called the American diet; which is red meat and sugar. This country gobbles down one meal after another of that red meat that is soaked with growth hormones, antibiotics, other drugs, chemicals from the food cows eat and parasites. Red meat increases the risk of cancer, heart disease, Alzheimer's, stomach ulcers and an array of other conditions. But this country just keeps right on scarfing down the red meat. And it's the main food for almost the entire country. The fat from red meat ends up clogging your veins and arteries. This fat along with vegetable oil is the major factor in creating clogged arteries and veins and raising blood pressure by accumulating on the walls of your veins and arteries. Once this plaque breaks off it can easily lodge in your brain or heart and cause a stroke or heart attack.

I got to tell you, it just bobbles the mind how we all stuff this garbage down our own throats and no matter how many consequences we suffer for doing so, we go right on doing it day after day to no end. Why? Because we refuse to face reality as it is. So we never even think corporations would be allowed to poison everyone for any reason, including the main reason most of these poisons are in your food, drinks and water - increasing corporate profits. Your life and health are irrelevant. We are not even human beings to the corporations. We are consumers, consumers of their products. And the only thing that means to corporations is that you are the ones they work to addict to their products.

And as long as you buy their products there is nothing they COULD do that would be wrong. NO WAY! Their poisons AND the products they use as the delivery device for those addicting poisons are FDA Certified safe.

All I can do is laugh at the extreme corruption of the FDA and the corporations. You need to re-evaluate your opinion of corporations who poison you in order to create changes in the human mind that cause your food addictions. As a matter of fact, all the food corporations are really doing is laughing all the way to the bank, while the medical industry laughs all the way to the bank too and thanks the food corporations for creating 75% of their business. They rake in the billions of dollars from you, while you suffer, lose your lives and end up bankrupt because of this transfer of wealth from you to the billion dollar corporations! And red meat is a major factor in all of this.

If dead cow flesh is as good for you as those who sell red meat claim, then why do you call dead cow flesh beef, steak, hamburger meat, hot dogs and all those other names substituted for dead cow flesh? It doesn't LOOK like they're trying to mislead, they ARE misleading you. Maybe if you would call something what it actually is, you might not be so quick to eat so much of it or not at all. And that's what's best for you. If you're going to eat dead cow flesh, I suggest you stick to Ground Chuck. Ground Chuck is ground beef without nearly as much fat. It's that fat, greasy taste you get addicted to eating red meat.

Now, I could go on about how bad red meat really is, but I've given you the information you need to make a rational decision to cut out red meat. If you can't cut out red meat now that you have faced the facts, then you are addicted to red meat. So to get off the red meat, you would have to pay attention to what's going on in your head while you are eating red meat. That's where the addiction is. And that's where you have to fight all these food addictions...in your head and way of thinking. Your body goes to work fighting all those chemicals and fat in red meat as soon as it gets into your body. And your body can't rid itself of those chemicals completely under normal circumstances.

So do yourself and your own health a big favor. Stop eating red meat! But since I know how hard it is to stop cold turkey, I recommend working to limit your red meat intake until you no longer eat red meat at all. I have already done this. But I do eat a pound or two of Ground Chuck in a pot of soup or a home cooked hamburger. I haven't eaten at McDonald's but once in the past 25 years, and that was when my wife and I were in Memphis for a major event. I have had my cholesterol checked and it is well within normal and I have no problems associated with cholesterol or fat. I hope you get off the red meat and the vegetable oils that are clogging your veins and arteries and disabling and killing tens of thousands of people every year in this country.

One other tip that can help is about outdoor charcoal grilling! I use to grill outdoors every few weeks until my kidneys blew out. But that all came to a screeching halt after that happened. I love eating charcoal grilled chicken, hamburgers, steaks, hot dogs and vegetable shishkabobs. But it's easy to see why it's all bad for you. First of all, it's bad enough that you're eating dead cow flesh. But on top of the meat already being drug saturated, you smoke it with burning charcoal!

Gee, why not just stuff a burnt wash cloth down your throat! Only difference would be the delay in taking your breath away and the time of death! Maybe you can just use the rule of doing these things in moderation and stop being so gung ho about stuffing as much red meat and charcoal grilled meat down your throat? Even the chicken, turkey and fish become repulsive to your body once they're heavily smoked on the outdoor grill.

So think about what you are really doing and stop lying to yourself about red meat being safe and smoking that meat being safe. Red meat is bad for you, and smoking it compounds that negative impact on your health. This country is obsessed with eating things that are very bad for you, while talking about the great food they are eating! This book seeks to cure you of that delusion and get you back on the road to healthy living and add days, weeks, months and years to your life and the lives of your family and other loved ones.

Vegetable oils – Canola Oil – Olive Oil or what? The simple answer to that question is olive oil. Olive oil is the best oil to use. But since it's quite costly it's not a practical solution for most people. Vegetable oils are always the cheapest. So people tend to lean heavily toward vegetable oils to cook with. But is your health and life really worth the savings in money? No it is not!

If you're old enough, you can remember how no one really said a thing about vegetable oils being bad for you until the past 20 years or less. But can you remember when no one thought cigarettes were bad for you either? Yea. **Doctors would go on TV and tell you not only that cigarettes were safe for you, but that cigarettes had quite a few health benefits.** Sounds crazy right? Totally crazy, right? It wasn't back then when they were doing this. There was no Public outcry against cigarettes at that time. People trusted their sorcerers with their new name "doctor", but not as much as people do now. They were pretty rational at that time, but were still tricked by the tobacco industry and the medical profession about cigarettes. And it's been the same story about vegetable oil and high fructose corn syrup.

You all choke down gobs and gobs of vegetable oils. It's bad enough that you cook in vegetable oil. But most of the vegetable oil you consume doesn't come from the foods soaked in vegetable oil that you fry at home. The biggest source of vegetable oils is in processed foods like Oreo cookies, Twinkies, potato chips, breads, cakes, pies, peanut butter and margarine! I'm not picking on just these food products. The grocery store shelves are packed with vegetable oil saturated food products just like the ones I just named. You need to look for trans-fat content on the label and avoid any products that have any trans-fats at all. In the ingredients, look for partially hydrogenated oils. Trans-fats are a byproduct which is created during partial dehydrogenation.

But beware! Just because the label lists trans-fats as zero, they can still have trans fats. Food manufacturers only list trans fats above zero if the product contains at least 0.5 grams of trans-fats per serving. They even fix the labeling per serving many times so they can claim their products contain zero trans-fats on the label. Trans-fats reduce the amount of good, HDL, cholesterol in your body. So if the ingredients list partially dehydrogenated oil of any kind, avoid that product. Do not buy it. But no matter how well you solve this problem in your own household, you still scarf down good amounts of vegetable oils when you eat any restaurant food.

There is no need to single out any one restaurant or many restaurants! Your whole problem with eating restaurant food is that none of it is healthy. They'll put out a salad bar at some places instead of cooking in Canola oil, using whole wheat flour, honey and no high fructose corn syrup. They are in business to make money and make as much money as they can within the Laws of this country. The problem is how we don't have a real government in this country any more. So it doesn't matter how bad these substances in the food supply are, as long as it's FDA approved, there is no government to do a thing about it.

Everything you eat in restaurants are cooked in vegetable oils. The damage those oils do to your body creates that craving for all the poison soaked foods and drinks you consume. It's that added taste that vegetable oils give foods that are cooked in vegetable oils. You think that chicken is good for you from that famous fried chicken restaurant, even though it's soaked in those artery clogging vegetable oils. Hey, I love their chicken. But I haven't eaten it but twice in the past four years.

About the only thing you can do about this is stop eating restaurant food; especially the big chain franchise restaurants. At smaller local restaurants you should tell the managers and owners of their restaurants that you want your food cooked in Canola oil and want a better choice of drinks with no high fructose corn syrup. Let them know it's a serious health need for you and your family. But don't let anyone distract you from your choices to avoid consuming foods and drinks that are bad for your health.

The only restaurant whose food I eat is almost always SubWay. I always get my sandwiches on multi-grain bread. I usually get the Orchard Chicken. It's like a chicken salad, but has cranberries, apple and black olives on it. Of course, you can get whatever you want on your sandwich, but cranberries are only on the Orchard Chicken that I know of. I also get the Oven Roasted Chicken as my second favorite, but sometimes will get a Philly Steak and Cheese or a Meatball sandwich. Although these sandwiches aren't as healthy as the Orchard Chicken, they come topped with lots of fresh sliced veggies. And having the multi-grain bread makes SubWay the healthiest restaurant eating I know of.

I might break down once every month or two and get a Veggie Lovers pizza from Pizza Hut, but Subway is easily our favorite restaurant. I like to eat some egg rolls from the Chinese restaurants too from time to time. But hey, eating out costs at least twice as much for the same food if you cook it at home. And with the very little chance of eating anything healthy from 99% of the restaurants, eating at home is the all-around best idea for sure. So eating at home is always going to be more healthy and cheaper than any food you can get in restaurants; especially the well-known fast food chains.

Olive oil is the best oil to use by far. Extra virgin olive oil is the best olive oil. Virgin olive oil is almost as good a quality as Extra Virgin Olive oil, but is not. I always buy Extra Virgin Olive oil for about $6 a quart. My wife uses olive oil to oil the skillet to cook grilled sandwiches and other light oiling cooking jobs. You can also whip up some mayonnaise using olive oil. It will last about 2 weeks in the refrigerator. Olive oil has many health benefits and has some great health care uses I bet most of you are unaware of! Always keep some olive oil in your home, and use it efficiently to make it go a long way. If money is no object, use it generously. The more you use olive oil, the better your health is going to be.

The best all-around oil is Canola oil. Although it doesn't have the extensive health benefits that olive oil has, Canola oil is about 25% the cost of Extra Virgin Olive Oil. Canola oil costs the same as vegetable oils. With that fact in mind, I can't understand why anyone would buy vegetable oil instead of Canola oil! There is no known damage which Canola does to your body. On the contrary! There are lots of people who take a tablespoon or two of Canola oil for their hearts most days. Canola oil has the lowest saturated fat content of all oils; including olive oil. It is very high in unsaturated fats too. Because of Canola oil's excellent health benefits, I suggest you read more about Canola oil and olive oil, and SEARCH the INTERNET too.

You do have to be careful when buying Canola oil, since 80% of the Canola oil made in this country is a GMO, Genetically Modified Organism. This is not true about Canola oil from outside the US, like Canada and Europe. Canola is really Canadian Low Acid Oil. Use expeller-pressed, non-GMO canola oil. I use very little oil for anything. So none of this is a concern to me. Just remember that almost all vegetable oils are GMO too. So Canola oil is the better choice.

Also, peanut oil has the most (good) mono unsaturated fat other than olive and Canola oil. Sunflower oil is also a better choice than vegetable oils, but still lags behind olive, Canola and peanut oil as far as overall health benefits. But it's still a much better choice than artery clogging vegetable oils. So avoid using vegetable oils by making the healthier choice at the grocery store. Stock up on it when it's on sale.

Sugars and Sweeteners – Now here's the information most people are interested in more than any other food information. It really does get confusing when you're trying to make healthy choices about sugar and other sweeteners. But just like all the food products we buy as consumers, healthy choices are hard to come by. Food companies are little to no help here either! The only healthy choices I know of among sweeteners is Stevia, raw honey and pure cane sugar. Since sugar is the most common sweetener by far, let's start there.

I told you to use pure cane sugar. But you have to pay attention to the precise term being used. You will often see, if not always, that white granulated sugar is called pure cane sugar. But it is NOT! Pure cane sugar is brown. Now you probably think you should buy brown sugar then, huh? Well don't! Brown sugar is just white granulated sugar sprayed with molasses. Brown sugar is not pure cane sugar as far as naming and labeling go. Confusing, right? Pure Cane sugar is named Pure Cane sugar and it is always BROWN. But Pure Cane sugar is not named or labeled as "brown sugar". **So you should only buy sugar that is brown not white and named "Pure Cane sugar".**

White granulated sugar is made by processing sugar cane. They remove everything that is good in the sugar cane and end up with white granulated sugar. During that process, they add sulfur dioxide, phosphoric acid and calcium hydroxide to the liquid cane sugar that eventually becomes white granulated sugar. White sugar is toxic to your body and weakens your body's ability to fight off disease. It also overloads your lymph system. Your lymph systems and nodes are part of your body's immune system. It's also a well-known fact that white granulated sugar causes tooth decay and is a major factor in obesity and diabetes. I have always referred to white granulated sugar as a drug, because that's what it is, pure poison that only harms your body.

Many others have started calling it a chemical. Your body sees it as a toxin that has to be removed. White granulated sugar, sucrose, has no real nutritional value. It only gives you empty calories. Those empty calories are high octane fuel inside your body. With all that sugar firing up inside your body as instant body fuel, energy, it should come as no surprise how that process is damaging your body inside or causing heartburn either. Scarf down white granulated sugar and heartburn is almost certain; and more so the older you get!

Avoiding white granulated sugar, sucrose, is a pretty humongous task in this country. The only consolation to consuming white granulated sugar is that it's not high fructose corn syrup. If you just gotta eat sweets, at least make sure it does not have high fructose corn syrup! White sugar is the lesser of two evils.

We have only bought one 4-lb bag of white granulated sugar in the past six years. We do buy the brown pure can sugar from time to time. Remember, brown pure cane sugar does still have the molasses in it and is the least processed of sugar cane sugars. So it is the healthiest of the cane sugars. If you just gotta continue with recipes that call for sugar, then substitute brown pure cane sugar for white sugar in your recipes.

There are a lot of restaurants that make their own ice cream using liquid pure cane sugar. You can tell it doesn't have that sugar bite you get eating white granulated sugar and high fructose corn syrup. Brown pure cane sugar will cost you more than white granulated sugar, even though it shouldn't! You're getting sugar that has no bad health consequences, besides all those calories, and that's the most important thing when it comes to what you eat and drink.

Sometimes you can find brand named Cokes, Dr. Pepper and others that use pure cane sugar instead of high fructose corn syrup. But none of them make a these products so you can buy them year round. I've bought root beer flavored sodas, like sarsaparilla, in natural food stores. I can tell the difference real well. But like all healthy products, they're hard to find. Healthy products will be hard to find as long as the food corporations continue to be obsessed with soaking their products with whatever poisons will addict you to their products the best.

Fructose is a better choice than white granulated sugar. Although fructose rhymes with sucrose, the name for white granulated sugar, fructose is twice as sweet per serving as sucrose. Fructose is not high fructose corn syrup either. Man-made unnatural fructose is bad for you though. I can only say there are healthier choices than fructose. You will find fructose in Gatorade. I keep seeing another derivative name for the sugar they put in Gatorade. So I backed off drinking Gatorade except for drinking some during hot weather.

Another familiar sweetener you see on products is Sucralose. Sucralose is the sweetener family name for a brand named product called Splenda. Although Splenda, Sucralose, is the least harmful of the man-made sweeteners, I don't use it. I don't use any of the artificial sweeteners. I have researched some other sweeteners, but haven't found any that I could trust. Aspartame is some bad crap! Some sources say that Aspartame turns to formaldehyde at about 80 degrees. I don't really know, even though it's very easy for me to believe that. I don't use Aspartame and would never recommend it. End of story.

Honey is another product that needs some precise information when you're buying it. You can't just pick any honey if you care about your health. You should only buy raw honey. Raw honey has not been processed. It takes honey a lot longer to start turning into a thick substance. Processed honey is always clear golden brown. Raw honey is golden brown too, but is cloudy instead of clear. Those beneficial bacteria in raw honey create this cloudiness.

Again, do your research into the many health benefits of raw honey, and do your INTERNET SEARCHes. It's hard to find raw honey in grocery stores. You should expect to pay $7 or $8 a quart when you do. I buy raw honey by the gallon for $26. It comes from a local bee farm. Use half as much raw honey as sugar if you substitute raw honey in recipes. Trying to sweeten your tea with raw honey is not really practical, although you can certainly do so if you can afford it. Use as much raw honey as you can afford. It's so good for you.

There is a host of things you can heal by taking equal amounts of raw honey and cinnamon, including - cancer, arthritis, pimples, heart disease, bad breath, cholesterol, colds, gas, bladder infections, restoring lost hearing and more.

When it comes to sweetening tea, we always use Stevia. Stevia is an herb that is about 30 times as sweet as sugar. Stevia has no calories too. Stevia also has no impact on diabetics, since Stevia does not affect blood sugar levels. So Stevia is an excellent healthy choice as a sweetener. When we make sweet tea at home, we use about 1/8 teaspoon per gallon of Lipton decaffeinated tea. We spend about $40 a year for enough Stevia to sweeten our tea.

I drink a lot of tea and I am thrilled to be doing so without swigging down all that white granulated sugar as I did for decades! What an improvement! If you have been sweetening your tea with sugar, tea sweetened with Stevia won't taste very good to you at first. You won't get that sugar bite or appease the addiction in your mind that happens to you from drinking sugar sweetened tea. So that makes you tend to think the Stevia isn't sweetening the tea very good and why your mind says it doesn't like it as well as sugary tea and drinks.

What you have to do to dispel this fallacy about the actual sweetness of Stevia is this: Make your tea as you always do. Before adding the Stevia, pour 2 or 3 ounces of the unsweetened tea into a glass. Then add the Stevia to the freshly made pitcher of tea and pour some of it into a glass. Drink the unsweetened tea, then the Stevia sweetened tea. You can tell the Stevia sweetened tea is sweetening the tea. But it's doing so without the harmful sugar bite you get from white granulated sugar, not to mention the case of "cotton mouth" you get from it! I love my Stevia sweetened tea. I did without tea after my kidneys failed, just to avoid all that sugar in liquid form. But thanks to Stevia I've been able to drink my tea AND not have any concern about the tea doing any harm to my health.

And one last thing - when I say you should drink plenty of water, that's doesn't include tea or anything that contains water. Drink all the Stevia sweetened tea you want. But don't count a bit of that tea as water.

Another sweetener you need to know about is Xylitol. Xylitol has 2/3 as many calories as white granulated sugar, but is safe for diabetics. Xylitol is found in a lot of fruits and vegetables in the fiber. Xylitol is a sugar alcohol. The most well-known use of Xylitol is for dental purposes. Xylitol kills the bacteria that cause gum disease and cavities. You will see it used in some sugarless gums too.

As a matter of fact, when I get a tooth ache the first thing I do is grab a couple of Xylitol mints and slide them around the affected area and let them dissolve. It helps a great deal every time. You can get Xylitol in gum or mint form, and in toothpastes.

Eggs – There's not a lot of choices when it comes to eggs. The USDA classifies eggs as meat due to their high protein content. Just because some eggs are brown doesn't mean they are healthier than white eggs. You have to make sure those brown eggs are actually organic eggs. To comply with USDA requirements to be able to label eggs as organic, the eggs have to come from chickens that have been fed organic feed, are free of antibiotics, as well as better standards for the welfare of the chickens.

The first thing you will find about the taste of organic eggs is how smooth they taste. Organic eggs don't have that chemical bite that regular eggs do. You will begin to recognize that chemical bite in regular eggs after you've eaten organic eggs for a few weeks. It's this chemical bite or burn that I focus on while I'm eating anything, in order to recognize how poisonous or healthy any food item is. I am extremely good at this.

There have been times when my wife bought some bad food product, and I used this ability and told her it has to have high fructose corn syrup. And sure enough, it does. It used to be hard for me to eat eggs. Even before I knew that bitter after taste was the chemicals in the eggs, I barely ate any eggs because of that. A better choice than regular eggs is Eggland Eggs. Eggland Eggs are organic eggs. These eggs come from chickens that are fed an organic vegetarian diet. For complete information on Eggland Eggs visit this web site –

http://www.egglandsbest.com/egglands-eggs/faq/our-eggs.aspx.

So far in this book I have touched on the tricks food corporations use to trick you into buying their products. Some of the most popular labeling scams are using terms such as Low fat, Low salt, Low Calorie, Organic, All Natural, Diet and From Concentrate. But as you'll find out, these terms are misleading and downright false as common sense goes. Take the Low fat, Low calorie and Low salt labeling scam. If a product contains all three of these ingredients and advertises one of these terms on the label, then the label is correct and legal. So no problem, right?

No, you are wrong! If a product label says Low Salt, but has sugar and fat in it too, the food companies add about twice as much sugar and fat as the regular version of the same product! But hey, at least they didn't lie on the label. They just didn't tell you on the label that it also had twice as much sugar and fat too! LOL You should read the label of the regular version of any product and compare it to the Low fat, Low calorie and/or Low Salt version of that product to confirm these facts. When I first started trying to avoid salt and sugar, I read hundreds of labels of products using these labeling terms and 100% of them confirmed these facts for me. I then ceased to buy any and all products with these labeling terms and so did some friends of mine.

So unless you have some specific condition that requires you to avoid salt, sugar or fat, then stick to buying the regular versions of these products. But make sure the regular version is a healthy choice or never put it in your grocery basket and bring it home. That's where **the front line on healthy eating and avoiding poisons is; right there in the grocery store reading those labels.**

Don't be fooled by other labeling tricks either, like Organic. I've pointed out some places you can trust the organic label term. But often times, organic doesn't mean organic. And it's left up to each one of us to sort this trickery out for ourselves. The same is true about the labeling terms Natural and All Natural. You also see the term natural ingredients as well, to convey a meaning of healthy food. But with all these terms, even the ingredients listed on the label itself will give you the proof to contradict these terms on most of these food and drink products.

You begin to find out what the food companies are pretending to be natural in their tiny world. Rare few of us would ever agree with the vast majority of the food and drinks corporations' idea of natural, All Natural and natural ingredients! **Just by using one of these new misleading label marketing tricks/terms, lots of you continue using unhealthy products.**

But in spite of all of this, you still have that wonderful fruit juice you love to drink. Yea, it's the one that says "Contains 100% Fruit Juice". I'm laughing now as I do just about every time I see that term on a product. If it's "100% Fruit Juice", then it contains ONLY fruit juice, right? Nope. Again, read the label and see if the juice is the only ingredient. If not, you have your proof about this misleading labeling term. When I see that term I always think "Yea, I bet you took a little bit of "100% Fruit Juice" and put it in that product. But what's all that other crap in there!"

Don't forget the whole wheat labeling trick where they call their products whole wheat by using white flour enriched with vitamins. Only buy those that say whole wheat flour or stoned ground whole wheat flour. Buy the brown pure cane sugar, not the white granulated sugar labeled as pure cane sugar. Don't be fooled by the new term for high fructose corn syrup, which is "corn sugar". They just changed the name, even though I had such wonderful (sarcastically saying) things to say about corn sugar under its real name – high fructose corn syrup. Like this:

It's just an adorable name...high...oh yes, I love to be high...fructose... ahh, it's SO SO SWEET...corn...yummy yummy corn...syrup...so thick and sweet, like me! Ba hum bug. Gag me with that poison and blow out my kidneys and almost kill me. Not so uplifting, yummy thick a product as the name implies. It should be called HFCS, Heinous Freakin' Causer of Sickness!

There has been lots of information about the negative effects of MSG, but food companies continue to use MSG. So you have to read the labels and do not buy products with MSG. Food manufacturers try to hide the fact that their products contain MSG by listing ingredients that contain MSG, but not the MSG itself. So avoid products if they contain free glutamate to insure your best possibility of avoiding MSG. Besides MSG, there are thousands of chemicals in food and drink products. My aim was to focus on how to reduce the total amount of poisons entering your body.

This is why I am not including a long drawn out explanation about the many other poisons in your food and drinks or in our water supplies and personal hygiene items. I have given you a powerful guide that will result in you reducing the amount of poisons getting into your body. **Remember, it's toxins, also known as free radicals and poisons, that cause almost all disease. So eliminating poisons is the action that reduces the amount of disease your body develops.**

I've even heard doctors state the fact that toxins, free radicals, cause many diseases. I just haven't ever seen a doctor with the desire to trace that toxin back to its source. As sad as it actually is, your doctor can't make money if he solves that problem; cures that disease by eliminating the poisons causing the disease or condition.

It's all up to each of you to use the power of knowledge in order to find your way through all the deceit that hurts us, but can't do a thing to change these food and drinks corporations. And that's what this book can do for you – to guide you through all the things that stand in your way, to keep you eating according to corporate advertising and misleading labeling, and the most important facts you need to make the serious changes concerning all the products you buy to consume. I will not suggest that you try talking with any of the food corporations or anyone in the government in pursuit of solving or diminishing this plague of poison induced sickness and disease affecting every human and animal in this country. Our humanity limits us time wise.

So use your time to read labels while you are in the grocery store. Work on recognizing the foods your mind craves when you are addicted to a food product. You have to understand that you can't wipe out all the poisons overnight! You have to start somewhere and keep learning progressively. Search the INTERNET for lots and lots of information on every subject and item. Look for information that repeats itself time after time while you're doing your searches and research. Cut back on eating out to avoid eating unhealthy. Cut down on charcoal grilling and the amount of meat you grill each time. The less poisons you put into your body, the less health problems you will have.

I also didn't spend time going over the details of the benefits of eating fresh fruits and vegetables. To me, that's real simple. Eat all the fresh fruits and vegetables you can. Just make sure you wash them real good. I even take each grape I eat and wipe it off real good with a paper towel.

To see for yourself what good this does, eat a few grapes and focus on the taste. Then wipe off a few grapes with a paper towel and eat them. Then eat some grapes without wiping them off and notice that slight bitter taste each grape has. That's the poisons the grapes are soaked in that you are tasting.

So wash all that fruit and vegetables extra good and eat all you want. And buy organic produce to reduce those poisons as much as possible. I'll even give you complete details on how to grow 100% organic produce later on in the book. And, Buy fresh over frozen, and frozen over canned.

Next are two chapters that are like chapters 5, 6 & 7, in that they should be a guide for your cures and preventions. Chapters 5, 6 & 7 guide you to read labels to avoid the poisons in your food, drinks and water. And chapter 8 is additional things you can do for specific diseases beyond the things everyone must do to lay the foundation for their cures. Chapter 9 gives you information about most of the Herbs, Vitamins and Healing Foods used in those cures. The heart of the information in this book are those chapters.

Wake up and get your attitude changed so you read labels as a way of life so you CAN avoid poisons. Let chapters 5, 6 & 7 guide you in cleaning up your current disease causing diet. Learn other things that help. And know what those vitamins, herbs and healing foods are and the science of how they help.

After all, wasn't it ME that told you to know what is in the things you eat, drink, bath and come in contact with!

8 -MORE Cures and Preventions

Here in this chapter is where you will find the specific information to speed your cures along for the conditions and diseases the modern medical profession in this country has no cures for. To them they are "incurable". The saddest fact about the medical profession is that they have led us all away from all the cures man has used in the entire history of the planet. This nationwide exodus away from the cures that man used throughout this planet's history began in earnest around 1939. I talked about this in detail in the chapter on the medical profession and health care system. We just simply need to get back to those cures and make them common knowledge among the people once again.

But even though these cures worked for man throughout history, they never had to deal with the huge amounts of chemicals that we all consume nowadays without thinking much about it. That's the major point of this book. You gotta face up to the facts about these poisons in your food, drinks and water; as well as your hygiene items. It's these poisons that cause most diseases and ailments; as much as 80% in my opinion and experiences.

There are two major areas you have to deal with and correct if you want to cure or prevent diseases. You have to work to get these poisons out of your life, AND you have to make sure you are giving your body what it needs and must have to keep you healthy and keep sickness at bay.

Your body uses its energy to digest food. When it's not digesting food, your body uses its energy to repair damaged cells. But your body also has to use energy to remove the poisons you put in your body. So all the poisons that get into your body use energy that could be being used to repair damaged cells. Fasting allows your body to spend all its energy removing toxins stored in the body and repairing damaged cells.

The key to curing your disease and any disease is learning to avoid poisons. I accidentally cured myself of every disease and condition I had by doing this, when I was only trying to help my kidneys get better.

If you want to speed your healing along, then do some fasting. When you fast, make sure you drink plenty of water; at least one ounce per two pounds body weight daily. A good fast is 3 days. But you can help yourself just by fasting for 12–16 hours as often as you choose. You could eat supper around 6 pm, then don't eat again until 6 AM or later. Fill your belly with cold water if you get hungry. Hippocrates, who is known as the father of medicine, based his practice on fasting and herbs; although modern medicine and doctors never prescribe or suggest fasting or herbs. I do the 12-16 hour fasts a lot.

I did fast for a week recently, but ate a bite of food here and there. I lost 12 pounds in that one week. I was only about 20-25 pounds overweight too. Check with your doctor about fasting if you have a serious disease or medical condition, if you want to fast more than 12-16 hours. It's sad that doctors betray their Hippocratic Oath by never prescribing fasting or herbs.

If you're looking for a miracle, then you will probably believe that you being cured of an incurable disease is indeed a miracle. **I wish I could revel in the glory of having brought your "miracle cures", but science isn't a miracle. Science can be explained. In the USA, we have drifted completely away from facts that use to be common knowledge among ourselves and others before us.** We think poisons are safe and don't hurt us any more, just because they're in our food and drinks and the FDA certifies them "safe"! But poisons are harmful. They always have been and always will be.

Get your head back on straight and get to working on ridding yourself of as much of these poisons as you can. You will get better at it as you go along. **But hear me loud and clear! Since these poisons cause most diseases, your disease will return with the return of the poisons that caused it in the first place. Be willing to make a lifestyle change to achieve your goals about your health**. So the only miracle going on here is the cure that is only a miracle because the medical profession has no cures.

The other major area in achieving a cure for your disease is correcting your diet deficiencies. The main problem with this is the fact that our food supply can't sustain good health for humans. I don't care how healthy you eat! The nutrients aren't in the growing fields to even have a chance to be in our food, even when it's "fresh". By the time a bell pepper, for example, gets to you it has lost up to 90% of its Vitamin C. And this is the case for all fresh produce. This is why you have to take vitamins. That was the reason I started taking vitamins at least 30 years ago. Because of this and other factors, we don't have much Magnesium in our diet.

Lack of Magnesium causes some serious problems such as bladder stones, kidney stones, bones spurs and heart arrhythmia That's why Magnesium cures bladder stones, kidney stones, bone spurs and heart arrhythmia.

But hey, if the doctor told you to take Magnesium instead of letting you suffer the rest of your life with bladder stones, the doctor wouldn't be able to make that money off you being sick. And since rare few people eat fish 2-3 times a week minimum as they should, pretty much everyone is Omega-3 deficient. Couple that with the high amounts of omega-6 in vegetable oils in so many products and your body and health takes a beating.

Since almost none of you get enough magnesium, Omega-3 and anti-oxidants, I have to advise EVERYONE to do the following, in addition to the things mentioned for any and all cures:

• **Take 250-400mg Magnesium oxide – 3000mg Fish oil and/or flax seed oil and 1000mg Vitamin C daily for 3-6 weeks. Then back off to just**

1000mg Fish oil and/or flax seed oil, but keep taking 1000mg Vitamin C and 250mg Magnesium every other day OR 2-3 times a week from then on. Fish oil and flax seed oil reduces all sorts of inflammation in your body.

• **In addition, you should take as many anti-oxidants as you can – Vitamin E, Vitamin A, Selenium and Alpha Lipoic Acid. A good dose of these would be 1000IU Vitamin E, 30,000IU Vitamin A and 200mcg Selenium daily or most days. These extra anti-oxidants will go a long way in removing toxins from your body.**

I didn't give you a dose for Alpha Lipoic Acid. Taking about 30mg to 50mg a day is OK. But always understand that Alpha Lipoic Acid causes your kidneys to reuse vitamins and nutrients 2-3 times. So if you are a kidney patient or have any other disease that calls for strict conformity of the amounts of Potassium or any other nutrient, then you may want to limit your Alpha Lipoic Acid and not take it more than 2 or 3 times a week. I took 600mg a day for 3 and a half months and it sent my Potassium above normal to 5.5. Once I stopped taking the Alpha Lipoic Acid, my Potassium went down to 4.7 within a few weeks.

Before we get to the specifics for cures, I want to remind you of how drinking pure water is the greatest thing you can do to improve your health. And the more you drink, the greater the benefit. So make those water filters your top priority on the path to curing yourself and preventing disease.

Get rid of the poisons while you follow these cures. And don't expect to cure yourself if you keep smoking cigarettes and/or drinking alcohol! They are both serious poisons. So don't play stupid and think you can keep smoking and drinking and still be cured. You've got to cut back on those things and get to where you can do without cigarettes and alcohol, at least until you are cured. After that, decide if going back to those poisons is worth the sickness it causes. It isn't! Good decision! If you must drink alcohol, then stick to no more than 2 ounces a day.

No matter what vitamins or herbs you take, never take any medications at the same time. Take any vitamins and herbs on an empty stomach, preferably before meals. Then take your drugs/medications after your meals. That way your food will be a buffer between the herbs and vitamins AND your drugs. You can also take your drugs OR vitamins and herbs, then take the other an hour later. So keep either a meal or an hour between doses of drugs, and vitamins and herbs.

Now I will list the diseases and conditions and give the cure and prevention for those diseases and conditions. And **remember, you do the things in this chapter in addition to drinking filtered water, baking soda, anti-oxidants, Magnesium and Omega-3 as the foundation for ALL these cures.** The information in this chapter is mostly additional things you can do to speed your cure along and is not a substitute for what I already said.

So, in alphabetical order here they are:

Acid Reflux – Commonly called **Heartburn**; acid reflux is caused by stomach acid flowing back up into your esophagus. This occurs when pressure or spasms cause the ring of muscles at the entrance of your stomach, called the lower esophageal sphincter (LES), to open too often or not close all the way. This produces that chest pain we call heartburn.

But what causes your stomach LES to do this? Just imagine putting a lid on a pot of boiling water, and how the boiling water and steam pop the lid up so some escapes. You put that high octane, high calorie, devoid of any nutritional value white granulated sugar or high fructose soda or fruit juice in your mouth, and it hits that stomach acid and kaboom!!!!!! The burning overflow is unavoidable. You need to alkalize your stomach and intestines AND stop gulping down the sugar and high fructose corn syrup in most foods and drinks.

While you are working to cure yourself of acid reflux by learning to recognize these poisons in products, you can cure your bouts of heartburn with baking soda and/or apple cider vinegar. Yep, apple cider vinegar. Unlike white vinegar, apple cider vinegar, ACV, is barely acidic. It is one of those natural foods like lemons and limes that turns alkaline in your body and neutralizes acid.

Just mix ½ teaspoon baking soda with 4-6 ounces of water and drink. This will stop your heartburn instantly. Drink baking soda and water 2x daily to keep from getting heartburn by raising the alkalinity of your body; which will also prevent almost all disease from having a chance to form. Disease cannot live in an alkaline body.

You can also drink 2 tablespoons of apple cider vinegar for your heartburn. I mix 2 tablespoons of apple cider vinegar with 2 teaspoons of raw honey, then add about 6 ounces of pure water and stir. It doesn't mix well, but the water and raw honey help take some of the edge off the apple cider vinegar. Your acid reflux will fade away within 2-3 months, and that purple pill the doctor prescribed you for the rest of your life will become obsolete.

Just think! Since 2 tablespoons of apple cider vinegar alleviates a bout of heartburn and only costs about THREE CENTS, how much money does that save you over the purple pill or ant-acids? And before you've used up a whole gallon of apple cider vinegar or less, your heartburn will be cured and gone. And it will stay gone until you give it back to yourself by eating more than a little bit of sugar, high fructose corn syrup and animal products. White flour and sugar in one product is a perfect recipe for instant heartburn too.

It is far better to use baking soda and/or apple cider vinegar for bouts of heartburn, but you can use TUMS too. I take TUMS, but not for heartburn. I take TUMS as an alkalizer, for general pH improvement. Aloe Vera is also a good alkalizer. Drinking aloe Vera juice is the preferred method; although aloe Vera capsules also help balance pH.

Alzheimer's Disease – You can cure your Alzheimer's and other brain diseases like Parkinson's and even strokes by following my advice for any other disease. That would be by taking 3000-5000mg Fish or Flax seed oil daily, 400mg Magnesium oxide, 3000-5000mg Vitamin C daily and drinking baking soda water at the rate of ½-teaspoon baking soda in 4-6-ounces water 3-5x daily. Plus, there are a host of natural things you can take to prevent damage to the brain which causes Alzheimer's. Drinking vegetable and fruit juices will do a lot toward curing your Alzheimer's; as well as some specific vitamins and herbs. I suggest you make your own juices from fresh fruits and vegetables to insure you are eating live food and not killing the life-giving enzymes in produce.

Some vitamins that help Alzheimer's include B Vitamins such as B6, folic acid and B12 which lowers homocysteine levels. High levels of homocysteine cause Alzheimer's to progress by causing neuronal damage in the brain. And higher levels of Vitamin B12 in your blood lower the risk of developing Alzheimer's. Taking anti-oxidants such as 100IU Vitamin E daily helps, as well as taking 10-50mg of Alpha Lipoic Acid daily. Niacin helps in reducing the severity of Alzheimer's. Acetyl L-Carnitine helps protect against amyloid-beta neurotoxicity when taken a few times a week at the rate of 100-300mg. Another valuable B vitamin is choline which is an acetylcholine precursor.

Some herbs which help people with Alzheimer's include Ginko Biloba and Curcumin. Curcumin is the yellow compound in Turmeric. Curcumin binds plaques and inhibits the formation of Abeta oligomers and fibrils. Sage is an herb that can help Alzheimer's because Sage contains cholinesterase inhibitors. Sage extract is the preferred form.

Taking anti-oxidants is real important since most Alzheimer's disease is caused by free radical damage to the brain over many years. Alzheimer's forms much faster if you have damage to your central nervous system. The brain is real sensitive to this oxidative damage by hypertension, diabetes and head trauma. These conditions cause a cytokine cascade and micro-localized inflammation in the central nervous system which results in Alzheimer's. So make sure you take Vitamin C, Alpha Lipoic Acid, Vitamin E and some other anti-oxidants as part of your cure and prevention for Alzheimer's.

Other things you should consider in your cure for Alzheimer's are Green Tea and other herbal teas, silica in your drinking water, Ginseng, DMAE, Tyrosine and Pantothenic acid. But do not forget to take Fish oil, since it contains good amounts of the fatty acid DHA. Doing so will greatly reduce the amount of beta-amyloid buildup in your brain that causes cognitive impairment.

Taking Lithium does three important things in the brain. It increases the size of the brain by promoting cell growth and slowing cell death and regeneration, protects against toxins that damage cells and nerve misfiring and helps form proteins that act as a shield to protect the brain.

Arthritis – Basically you need 3000mg Fish oil and 1500mg Glucosamine daily for 4-6 weeks, followed by a few months of 1000mg Fish oil and 1000mg Glucosamine daily. After that, take a maintenance or preventative dose of 1000mg Fish oil and 1000mg Glucosamine 2 or 3 times weekly. Your arthritis will fade away and go away completely. You can also substitute flax seed oil for some of the Fish oil. The Fish oil provides you with Omega-3 and lubricates your joints, while Glucosamine builds the cartridge that cushions and pads your joints. This combination cures your arthritis. And Fish oil and flax seed oil are both anti-inflammatory for reducing and eliminating inflammation in the body. MSM also aids in preventing and curing arthritis, as well as relieving joint pain and inflammation. MSM builds tissue in your cartridge and improves allergies, asthma and digestive tract problems. I have tried Chondroitin, but do not use it. It's far too expensive for the small benefit it may bring.

Back Pain & Problems – I have suffered with back pain from time to time. I always know what caused it too. DUH! There are a lot of things you can do to help ease and prevent back pain. The easiest way to do this is to get an Inversion table and an AB Chair or similar AB machine. An inversion table does something that you can hardly do once you become an adult. It allows you to hang upside down like you did as a kid on the monkey bars in elementary school. An Inversion table straps your ankles onto a stretcher so that you can hang by your ankles. What this does is reverse the effects of gravity on your body and spine. Gravity is pushing down on your body 100% of the time.

You have to suspend your body by the ankles to get gravity to reverse the effects of gravity when standing upright. Hanging on an Inversion table helps align the spine and take pressure off your spinal discs, and causes blood to rush downward into your chest, head and neck. This brings better blood circulation to the upper body and head, and gives you a refreshing feeling. I have used an Inversion table for at least 20 years. And when my back hurts, I always hang on the inversion table a few minutes 3 or 4 times a day. An inversion table helps reverse the constant downward force 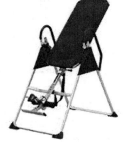 gravity exerts on your body. Back pain is also caused by weak back muscles.

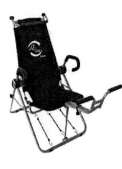 For weak back muscles use an AB Chair. They also have different brand names like AB Lounger and such. But it's a canvas chair on a metal frame that you do sit ups on. Using an AB Chair or doing regular sit ups will go a long ways in strengthening back muscles and preventing back pain. A too soft mattress will create back pain in your lower back and hips. We have to take our memory foam off our bed for months at a time when I get lower back pain. Once we do that, my lower back pain goes away within 2-3 days.

To relieve lower back pain you can also do this stretching exercise: Sit on the floor with your back against the wall and slide your back and butt up against the wall firmly with your legs stretched straight out from your body. Then take your right foot and place the bottom arch of your foot sideways against the side of your left knee and hold that position. Do the same thing placing your LEFT foot against the side of your RIGHT knee. This brings temporary relief every time.

I also use what is called a Spine Aligner. It is a piece of molded plastic with two rubber cushion strips to cushion the edges of the molded plastic that cushions your back as your spine falls in the long groove, to be forced back into alignment by the natural force and weight of your body.

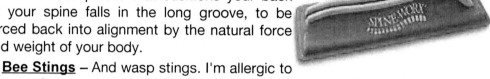

Bee Stings – And wasp stings. I'm allergic to bees and wasps, so I swell up big time when I get stung. I never knew much of anything you can do for a wasp or bee sting, or didn't know until I tried rubbing an onion on the sting. I had heard about this somewhere in the past, but had never had a chance to test it until about 10 years ago. My wife got stung by a wasp and when nothing helped, I thought of the onion thing. I cut off the end of a yellow onion and grabbed it by the tail all onions have and rubbed the fresh raw onion on my wife's wasp sting. Within 15 minutes the swelling went all the way down and stayed down. Plus, the sharp stinging pain went away too.

I did the same thing for myself when I got stung inside my house by a wasp and my wife stepped on a bee in the yard. The onion did the trick all three times. I was really shocked since, as I told you, I'm allergic to bees and wasps. A sting is a 2 or 3 day ordeal for me. But not after using the onion. Applying raw honey to a sting will help quite a bit too.

Bladder Stones - To cure bladder stones you need to understand how bladder stones form. Bladder stones are formed by particles of calcium combining with toxins to form those prickly stones. So you have to deal with both the calcium particles and the toxins to cure bladder stones. Calcium needs Magnesium to dissolve it to make calcium ready to be used by the body. If you don't have enough magnesium, then calcium is available to bind with toxins, free radicals, to form bladder stones, kidney stones and bone spurs.

So taking 250-400mg Magnesium will take care of that. But, you still have to take anti-oxidants to rid your body of toxins. Vitamin C will go a long ways, but you need to take as many anti-oxidants as you can, to do a thorough job against toxins. So take Vitamin E, Vitamin A, Selenium and some Alpha Lipoic Acid. 1000mg Vitamin C and 250mg magnesium is the least you need daily.

If you already have bladder stones, then take 250-400mg twice daily. Taking an excess of Magnesium will provide your body with the Magnesium it needs to make you healthy and the extra Magnesium to erode and dissolve those bladder stones, kidney stones and bone spurs. I always tell people how natural cures take weeks to a few months. But my own experience proved that when it comes to bladder stones you can be cured instantly. When I had my fourth bladder stone attack, I did not go to the hospital again. I took two 250mg Magnesium oxide tablets. And less than an hour later the attack stopped and I haven't had one attack in the seventeen years since then. I still take 250mg Magnesium 2-3 times a week to make sure they never come back.

Bone Spurs – The cure for bone spurs is the same as the cure for bladder stones and calcium based kidney stones. See above. **Also, remember to start your dogs on the preventative dose at age 6, since bone spurs and/or bladder stones is a sure thing for almost all dogs, if not all dogs. Every dog I've had that lived beyond age 8 had either bladder stones or bone spurs.**

Breast Cancer - It's a scientific fact that flax seed oil kills breast cancer cells at least as fast as chemical therapy, but without all the pain, suffering, hair loss and huge medical bills as the medical profession's artificial chemotherapy. If you had been on a proper human diet of fish, you most likely wouldn't have gotten breast cancer in the first place. The Omega-3 fat, alpha-linolenic acid, found in flax seed, walnuts and cold water fish like tuna and salmon, provide the best protection against breast cancer. Studies have shown that women with higher Omega-3 content in their breasts had the lowest risk of breast cancer.

It's pretty much common knowledge that a woman's breast is mostly fatty tissue. And with all the omega-6 rich vegetable oils you consume combined with the low levels of Omega-3 in the normal red meat American diet, that throws the healthy ratio of omega-6 to Omega-3 fats way out of ratio. This creates a disease ripe environment for breast cancer and other cancers. Add to that, all the poisons you have yet to recognize and avoid, is it any wonder why you have breast cancer!

Since many breast cancers depend on estrogen, you should take Calcium D-Glucarate; which helps the body excrete used hormones such as estrogen. Calcium D-Glucarate is known to remove, detoxify, cancer causing carcinogens in the colon, skin, liver, breasts and lungs. Do not confuse Calcium D-Glucarate with any other form of calcium. Buy only products that state the term Calcium D-Glucarate clearly and specifically. Calcium D-Glucarate is found in many fruits and vegetables, but one 500mg tablet of Calcium D-Glucarate contains as much phytonutrient as 82 pounds of fresh fruit and vegetables.

And don't forget the anti-oxidants either. Vitamin C, A and Selenium to remove toxins and Vitamin E to help speed along healing of damaged cells.

Cancer – *This is a brief summary of the information in Chapter 10 – The Cure For Cancer.* Cancer is caused by damage to the nucleus of cells. This damage interferes with apoptosis, which is the natural programmed death of cells. When this process breaks down, cancer cells begin to form. Cancer cells do not experience programmed death as normal cells do. This allows cancer cells to grow and divide; which leads to a mass of abnormal cells that grows out of control and forms tumors. Once these tumors form, they develop blood vessels. These blood vessels carry cancer cells to other parts of the body and form growths.

The damage to cells is caused by gene mutations causing cells to be unable to correct DNA damage. Cancer is a result of these mutations which interfere with oncogene and tumor suppression gene function and leads to this uncontrollable cell growth. Carcinogens are directly responsible for damaging DNA and promoting cancer. Free radicals are formed when our bodies are exposed to carcinogens. These free radicals damage cells and inhibit normal cell function. If your family members have had cancer, especially your parents and grandparents, it's obvious this gene mutation was passed on to you.

But even so, this only means cancer forms quicker in these people than those without the family history of cancer. And as soon as your body is exposed to carcinogens, cancer begins to form.

So, you can easily see how **avoiding poisons is the key to preventing and curing cancer. This is why all cancer patients should get serious about avoiding and eliminating poisons, like I have laid out in this book.** You should avoid smoking and excess exposure to the sun. Since free radicals cause cell damage, you should take all the anti-oxidants you can. Take the prevention/maintenance dose if you don't already have cancer. If you already have cancer, take mega doses of Vitamin C. A mega dose would be at least 5000mg daily and as much as 10,000mg daily.

Also double the maintenance dose of Vitamin E, A and Selenium and take around 100mg of Alpha Lipoic Acid most days to boost the effectiveness of those anti-oxidants. Take Fish oil and/or flax seed oil too, as recommended at the beginning of this chapter; since both are anti-inflammatory and help create balance with omega-6 to prevent and cure disease.

Your immune system controls cancer cells in your body. You rarely have a problem with cancer as long as your immune system is healthy. Your immune system works to remove toxins to keep you healthy. Take Astragalus and even dandelion root to boost your immune system. Take 1000-3000mg daily for 2-3 weeks, then 1000mg Astragalus every other day or every few days as a maintenance dose.

As you may recall, I pointed out earlier in this book that sodium benzoate and high fructose corn syrup cause DNA damage. So anything with either of these should be high on your list of poisons to eliminate. Soda pops have both of these poisons. And much to my surprise, Mrs. Weavers sandwich spreads have sodium benzoate. So we rarely ever buy Mrs. Weavers pimento, chicken or ham sandwich spreads. I always loved her products too. This is why you read the labels before buying any product. It takes valuable time out of our busy lives, but is THE KEY in avoiding products with these poisons. Don't make the mistake I did, and do this AFTER you are already sick.

Which would you choose? Having cancer and wishing you had've taken the time to read the labels and avoided getting cancer or some other disease? OR Taking the time to read the labels and avoid the cancer altogether? **Living this chronic delusion that poisons are safe as long as they're in our food, drinks, hygiene items and water supplies is the problem this book cures. Once this problem is solved so that poisons are bad for you, especially when those poisons are in your food, drinks and water, disease will fade to the background** and most of us can die like most people use to, of old age; not disease. And cancer will cease taking our loved ones prematurely!

I am always amazed at how even though toxins, aka poisons and free radicals, cause cancer, I haven't heard about any doctor telling anyone to get rid of the poisons that caused their cancer. That is, beyond saying to stop smoking! But you can keep right on obeying your doctor and paying those high medical bills WHILE you cure yourself naturally and without all that suffering and pain.

Colds and Flus – Yes, there has always been a cure for the common cold and a preventative. These facts are so damning of the modern medical profession. A strong immune system is the key to preventing disease. But to put it simply, to prevent colds, in August start taking 1000mg of Vitamin C as cold and flu season approaches. Keep this up all through the cold and flu season to prevent colds and flus. If you already have a cold, then take 1000mg Vitamin C every 4-6 hours until you are well; usually 3-4 days later instead of 10-14 days or more. Boost that Vitamin C with at least 100mg Alpha Lipoic Acid daily while sick or even as much as 300-600mg.

Also take Echinacea to help kill germs and viruses. Studies show Echinacea can cut your chances of getting a cold in half. Take Astragalus to boost your immune system. Take 400mg of Echinacea every 4-8 hours daily and 1000mg Astragalus 3 times daily. But only take 400mg Echinacea and 1000mg Astragalus daily as a maintenance, preventative dose. Taking other anti-oxidants will also aid in the prevention and cure of common colds and flus.

Monolaurin, or monolauric acid, interferes with a virus cell's ability to reproduce. So Monolaurin is taken for the flu and colds. Monolaurin is found in breast milk and is a major factor in boosting a baby's immune system. Commercial Monolaurin is derived from bitter melon, coconuts or saw palmetto.

These same things will help you cure yourself of the flu. I say that and yes it's true. But people have been getting some strange flus the past couple of years. So I advise you to seek medical help from a doctor or ER if your flu symptoms are not normal flu symptoms; such as is the case with swine flu.

Constipation and other Colon problems – Your first act would be to choose a colon cleanser and use it. To choose which one you want, this web site can help you with that – www.detoxreviews.com. I have used Almighty Cleanse and Colonix. Both are pretty good products. You want to look for that snotty looking stuff hanging from your poop when you use any colon cleanser.

A good colon cleanser will loosen that snotty greenish mucus that forms on the walls of your intestines. This mucus forms to protect your intestines from the poisons you consume. Pockets of feces form in your large intestines, but should come out by doing a good cleanser.

You can have as much as 15 pounds of fecal matter in these intestinal pockets. These conditions also cause bloating and weight gain; not to mention the fact that your body can't absorb nutrients very well with your large intestine coated with mucus. And that poop lodged in your intestine walls rots for long periods of time!!! A good colon cleanse and lots of pure water and fresh fruits and vegetables will make that colon cleanser work much much better. And it will cure that constipation too.

Probiotics should be part of any colon cleansing package. And you should continue using probiotics from time to time after your colon cleanses. I use and recommend **Dr. Ohhira's Probiotics 12 Plus** and **ThreeLac**. ThreeLac kills candida overpopulation in the intestinal tracts.

But if you want to avoid constipation, you have to get fiber in your body. The easiest way is to eat fresh fruits and vegetables, whole wheat, other whole grains, brown rice and even frozen fruits and vegetables and dried fruit & nuts.

Dandruff, dry skin and dry hair – To cure dandruff, dry skin and dry hair, you need to buy and install a shower water filter. I had dandruff for most of my life; sometimes more than others. I tried many different medicated shampoos, but none ever really solved the dandruff problem. I also use to get dry red itchy spots on my body after taking a shower. I made all kinds of excuses about what might be causing those red itchy places. I blamed the weather and other things. I bought a shower filter when I first got serious about eliminating poisons to try and help my kidneys. Three weeks after I got the shower filter, those dry red itchy places had disappeared.

My years of dandruff all but ended about that time too. It turns out that the chlorine in the water was responsible. Chlorine destroys the oils in your hair and skin. So natural science was causing my dandruff and red itchy dry spots on my body. It's time to get that shower filter, right!

One thing you can do for your dry skin and hair is use Extra Virgin Olive oil. Yes, that's what I said - Extra Virgin Olive oil! I have found that using Extra Virgin Olive oil does the best job of healing dry skin and hair. Simply apply the Olive oil straight out of the bottle, same as you would any lotion or shampoo. You may want to apply Olive oil to your hair and scalp right before you go to bed. When you get up in the morning, wash it out. You will be amazed at how soft your hair is! Same thing goes for your dry skin.

All those years of dandruff and the cause was the chlorine in the shower water! My dandruff went from a snowfall to a speck here and there when I scratched my scalp. You won't see any white flakes on MY black shirts! And those red itchy dry places never came back. They're just a memory now!

Diabetes – There are two major things you have to know to prevent or cure diabetes. You know you have to try and avoid sugar. But your pancreas also helps you to digest your food. **The amount of pancreatic secretions depends on how well you chewed your food and covered each bite with saliva.** To help take the load off your pancreas, take digestive enzymes such as papaya enzyme and Bromelain. Bromelain is especially good at aiding in the digestion of protein. I take it every time I eat meat; and take papaya enzyme for everything else.

If you don't chew your food up real good, then it is up to the stomach to break the food down. If after about an hour and a half, your stomach hasn't broken down all the solid pieces, your pancreas releases enzymes to do so. But if you chew each bite of your food to get it covered in saliva and to make the food much easier for you to digest, then you will significantly reduce the amount of work your pancreas has to do to help digest whatever you consume.

Some things you have to remember when attempting to avoid sugar are: Avoid high fructose corn syrup. It's a far worse factor in diabetes than any sugar. Never eat sugary foods or drinks on an empty stomach. Doing this allows maximum and quickest rate of absorption into your system. Try sticking to safe alternatives to sugar, like raw honey and Stevia; and if necessary, use Splenda. Don't ever drink any juice unless it says "Not From Concentrate" or "Never From Concentrate".

Taking 500mg of Taurine 3 times a day will help your pancreas. Taurine acts as a powerful antioxidant for your pancreas, to neutralize the destructive effects of oxygen free radicals. Taurine improves insulin resistance too.

Taking Bilberry helps promote healthy blood sugar levels and healthy insulin production. Magnesium also helps regulate blood sugar levels. Cinnamon does such a good job of controlling blood sugar levels, some people take cinnamon in place of insulin. It really is that good in the cure and prevention of diabetes.

Take GTF chromium. GTF stands for Glucose Tolerance Factor. **Do not take chromium picolinate. Only take chromium that is clearly specified as GTF Chromium.** Men should take 400-600mcg per day and women 200-400mcg daily. GTF chromium is named for the way it interacts with insulin to improve the body's sensitivity to insulin. GTF chromium also improves your blood lipids profiles for triglycerides and LDL cholesterol (bad cholesterol).

Erectile Dysfunction - Viagra is used to treat the symptoms of erectile dysfunction. But you need a cure for it. I was shocked that one of the blood pressure medications had caused me to temporarily develop this condition. Doctors suggested testosterone shots and salve. But I decided to seek out a natural cure. I soon ran across an herb called Tribulus Terrestris. It doesn't actually produce any testosterone. But Tribulus Terrestris stimulates the production of LH, luteinizing hormone; which causes the natural production of testosterone. And instead of using Viagra while you are curing yourself, you can use Horny Goat Weed. I cured the E.D. within 2-3 months; as well as another physical problem caused by low testosterone and high estrogen.

Eye disease - Bilberry (Vaccinium myrtillus) contains nutrients that protect eyes from eye strain or fatigue and can improve circulation to the eyes, improving the micro circulation and regeneration of retinal purple; a substance required for good eyesight. Bilberry helps produce anthocyanosides which support and enhance the health of collagen structures in the blood vessels of the eyes; thus aiding in the development of strong healthy capillaries that can carry vital nutrients to eye muscles and nerves. Bilberry has long been a remedy for poor vision and "night blindness." Bilberry tends to improve visual accuracy in healthy people and can help those with eye disorders such as pigmentosa, retinitis, glaucoma, and myopia.

Two other substances that help the eyes are Lutein and Vitamin A. Vitamin A helps prevent or slow macular degeneration. Lutein is a powerful antioxidant that protects our eyes from free radical damage; which play a major role in the development of macular degeneration and cataracts. Lutein also protects the macula from blue and ultraviolet light. The macula is responsible for our central vision and sharp detailed vision.

Try taking 30,000IU Vitamin A, 1000mg Bilberry and 20-40mg Lutein daily.

Fibromyalgia – The one thing I know that will help fibromyalgia is taking a product called Corvalen. Corvalen is D-Ribose. D-Ribose helps your body produce ATP; which is an energy cell. The main energy cells in your body, like ATP, are made of ribose, plus B vitamins and phosphate. So ribose, sold as Corvalen, brings relief to those suffering with fibromyalgia or chronic fatigue syndrome. But of course, fibromyalgia is caused by toxins in your body. Although I can't confirm that Corvalen cures you, I know it does give you relief from fibromyalgia and CFS. Use Corvalen, exercise, stretch, drink lots of pure water and work on avoiding the poisons this book points out, and I think you may just cure yourself. I included this information about fibromyalgia as a help, not a cure. But this may very well cure you too.

Gout – Gout is an extremely painful condition. Gout is caused by an overproduction and over population of uric acid. Uric acid has needle-like points on the crystals. The pain of gout is caused by those needle-like crystals. Just imagine tens of thousands of needles inside your big toe or ankle, and you get the idea behind what gout is doing to you. Although most gout attacks are the result of consumption of high fructose corn syrup, especially in liquid form such as fruit juices and soda pops, gout is also caused by other things.

The common factor among all the causes is the introduction of poisons or some other body trauma such as chemotherapy, joint injury and dehydration. This tells you that drinking lots of pure water will help gout. And working on avoiding poisons in your food and drinks will cure your gout, and/or prevent gout altogether. Drinking too much alcohol can bring on a gout attack. Alcohol is mostly a sugar, and a poison to your body. Drinking beer and eating shrimp together are known to cause gout.

I cured myself of gout by getting off the high fructose corn syrup. And I nailed this fact down forever. I went through a phase for 2 to 3 months where I was tired of being laughed at and hated on because of my speaking out against high fructose corn syrup. So, I just gave it up and decided that since I'm so crazy for speaking out against high fructose corn syrup, I would now shut my mouth and never do it again. And since, according to most everyone else, high fructose corn syrup is only a poison in MY crazy opinion, then it was perfectly safe for me to consume high fructose corn syrup.

I stopped trying to avoid high fructose corn syrup for 2-3 months. Then I got gout again, and had gout all day every day for TWO WHOLE MONTHS! And that is what broke me and stood me up against high fructose corn syrup FOREVER! I mean this one is nailed down! But, to test this "opinion" of mine one final time, I told myself I would stay off the high fructose corn syrup, UNLESS I had another gout attack AFTER getting off the high fructose corn syrup again. It's been 2 years since that last gout attack, so I know it's the high fructose corn syrup. That was the main factor in making my body acidic.

Drinking baking soda water and adding pH drops to my drinking water were the other two things I did to finally end my gout. But you really need to work on avoiding poisons, as this book explains, and do things to boost your immune system like taking Astragalus. Avoiding aluminum based anti-deodorants will help too, by keeping your lymph system healthy. Once that aluminum soaks into your underarm, it poisons your lymph glands and nodes. Your lymph system is part of your immune system.

If you just have to use drugs, ask your doctor to prescribe you Colchicine. It is taken when you feel a gout attack coming on. Otherwise, you'll be taking gout medication every day to prevent gout until you can get yourself completely cured. But to make sure you cure gout, drink baking soda water at the rate of ½ teaspoon per 4-6 ounces water 2-5x daily until cured.

Baking soda is alkaline and gout is sharp Uric acid crystals with needle-like points on every one of them. Alkaline substances neutralize acid. So this easy low cost cure for gout is easy to see and understand. This also cures Uric acid kidney stones, which are much harder to cure than calcium based stones.

Gums bleeding – This is another disease that I cured myself of just by waging war against high fructose corn syrup and other poisons. My gums had turned to mush over the years and bled every time I brushed my teeth. I can look back and get a good picture of what my kidneys had done - turned to mush. Since getting off the high fructose corn syrup, my gums stopped bleeding every time I brush my teeth, as they had done the past 10-20 years.

But just as other chronic conditions faded away and never came back, so did my bleeding gums. All because of me getting off the high fructose corn syrup and other poisons! My gums haven't bled but once since they stopped 6 years ago. And my gums have firmed up around my teeth nicely.

Use salt water to clean and soothe your gums, especially when you have tooth pain. Use hydrogen peroxide to stop bleeding in your gums or any place else. Brushing with just 4-5 drops of tea tree oil will soothe gums and kills germs as well as antibiotics do. It tastes like turpentine, but works great. Xylitol does just as well. Use Clove oil or Cinnamon on your gums to relieve pain.

Brushing with baking soda goes a long way in ending bleeding gums too. The high pH of the baking soda neutralizes the acids that cause tooth decay, rots your gums and is behind almost all toothaches. Just wet your brush with water. Shake off any excess water and dip your toothbrush in baking soda and brush your teeth. Make sure you do this before bed so you have all that acid in your mouth neutralized for the 8 hours you are asleep.

Headaches – Again, I cured myself of at least 20 years of regular headaches of about 4 to 5 days a week. I had just gotten use to taking Ibuprofen, Tylenol and aspirin to relieve those headaches. So that's all I did for my headaches until the end of 2006. **Using the information in this book, I reduced the amount of poisons and the end of my headaches was among the diseases to be cured. Those Ibuprofen are hard on your kidneys too. I have not had any headaches since early 2007. I credit getting off the high fructose corn syrup as THE main reason for that.** Even eating too much sugar can give you a headache; especially if you pile that sugary desert on top of a meal.

Make sure you follow my instructions at the first of this chapter about taking magnesium, Fish oil and anti-oxidants. Toxins cause those headaches, so take antioxidants. Headaches are also caused by tension, and Magnesium helps to relax muscles. Fish oil is known to help diseases of the brain, and raises levels of an enzyme that protects brain cells from plaque buildup. Fish oil supplies DHA to improve brain functions too. All these help bring an end to headaches.

Heartburn – See **Acid Reflux**

Heart disease – Basically, you need to take Magnesium and Fish oil. Flax seed oil is also good for the heart. Your heart needs calcium to contract and Magnesium to relax your heart. This produces normal heart rhythms. Take 250-

400mg daily for a few weeks if you haven't already been taking Magnesium tablets. Then go to a maintenance dose of 250-400mg daily or every few days.

Co-Q10 helps make your veins and arteries more elastic, which helps cure hardening of the arteries. Fish oil produces the same effect by emulsifying the fats and plaque that build up in your arteries and promote atherosclerosis. Take 100-150mg Co-Q10 daily and at least 1000mg fish or flax seed oil daily. Fish oil and flax seed oil help your heart and blood pressure because they contain Omega-3 fatty acid. Fish oil helps improve circulation. Omega-3 also reduces sudden death from cardiac arrhythmias. Fish oil also reduces triglyceride levels and helps stabilize blood clotting mechanisms which prevents blood clots; a major cause of heart attacks and strokes. Fish oil "thins" the blood.

Niacin helps clean plaque and other debris in your blood, veins and arteries. Taking Fish oil and niacin can cure heart disease caused by plaque and hardening of the arteries. You need to take large doses of niacin to do this. But you run into a peculiar problem known as the red flush. Red flush is caused by doses of niacin as low as 25mg. This red flush is caused by the niacin expanding your capillaries to twice their normal size; allowing more blood flow to the surface of the skin. Be glad when you get it! This is the proof of the niacin working. By expanding your capillaries, your blood is able to carry a lot more toxins out of your body. To increase your dose of niacin, do this:

Start with 25mg niacin 2-3 times a day. When you no longer get the red flush, increase the dose to 50mg 2-3 times a day. Repeat this until you are at 100mg 2-3 times a day. Then up the dose by 50mg each time until you no longer get the red flush. You can do this all the way up to 500mg. Just remember that if you stop taking niacin for a while, don't start back taking the same dose as you were. The red flush could very well be painful instead of slightly uncomfortable.

When I was first diagnosed with chronic kidney disease, my EKG showed that I had an enlarged heart. I had trouble breathing more than a few times in those months just prior to and after that EKG. Doctors only expected it to get worse, not better. Because of the way I have eaten the past 30 years, I don't have a problem with cholesterol. But I cured myself of an enlarged heart by doing the same things I told you here and getting rid of the poisons I was consuming. I asked Dr. Allen if I could get another EKG to see if I had damaged my heart by having long term high blood pressure. My EKG was very good, and a few months after that I had an EKG done again. It was almost perfect.

Be sure to read the cure for **Stress** to help minimize putting harmful pressure on your heart and circulatory system. And of course, exercise regularly, drink lots of pure water and eat as many fresh fruits and vegetables as you can. And, since people often mistake heartburn (acid reflux) as a heart attack, be sure to follow the instructions for **Acid Reflux**.

Cardiovascular disease is the leading cause of death in the USA, even though almost all heart disease is preventable. Use this book to help you do so.

Intestinal bleeding - stomach ulcers – Intestinal bleeding is usually caused by high fructose corn syrup, sugar and white flour burning your intestines until it begins to bleed. This is easy to do since years of drinking chlorinated water has killed most of the beneficial bacteria in your digestive tract. So, the more you avoid high fructose corn syrup, sugar and white flour, the sooner your bleeding ulcers go away.

To replenish the beneficial bacteria that chlorinated water kills, take probiotics. Also, doing a colon cleanse will remove the mucus from your intestinal walls and remove impacted feces. These conditions promote intestinal bleeding. I have noticed the link between heartburn and intestinal bleeding. Both are pretty much caused by the same things; just in different parts of the body. Heartburn occurs above the stomach in the throat and esophagus, and "heartburn" in the intestinal tract produces bleeding ulcers. Take cayenne, garlic and sage to ease and cure your bleeding ulcers and repair your stomach and intestinal walls.

Kidney disease – The most complete information for curing kidney disease is found in chapter 11. This is a summary of things you can do to cure kidney disease. So make sure you read chapter 11 if you have any kind of kidney disease. It's a disease I know a whole lot about. Everything I did the past 5 years was centered around my chronic kidney disease. I have tried all kinds of things. Most of them helped. A few did not help.

The best thing for kidney disease is pure water. So start with a fluoride water filter as I pointed out in the Poisons in Your Water chapter. Drink 1 ounce of water for every 2 pounds of body weight. Drinking water is the best way to wash and cleanse your insides. But drinking water with chlorine and fluoride is almost enough to negate the positive effects water has on your kidneys and whole body. So at least get a carbon water filter to filter out 90% of the chlorine and no fluoride! They only cost $20-30.

Making sure you hold your blood pressure down is essential, and your doctor will tell you this. Take Hawthorn berries, L-Arginine, Fish oil, magnesium, B6 and garlic to help lower your blood pressure naturally, in addition to your prescribed medicines. Even apple cider vinegar can lower your blood pressure. It's high in vitamins that are helpful for lowering blood pressure, like Vitamins C, A, E, B1, B2 and B6, as well as Potassium, Magnesium and copper.

Apple Cider Vinegar is alkaline, so it improves your body's pH levels. See **Acid Reflux** for how to use ACV. Valerian Root helps to calm you and lower blood pressure, but should be taken with caution and only according to directions. Dealing with stress goes a long way in controlling your blood pressure. So make sure you follow the instructions on curing **Stress.**

It is my opinion that you are best off taking Clonidine and Quinapril to control blood pressure artificially. Taking Atenolol only slows down your heartbeat to minimize the number of times your heart beats, but doesn't actually lower your blood pressure. You could also take a CCB, Calcium Channel Blocker, but only do so for about a year at a time, since doing so any longer may weaken your bones, as told later. Due to the damage to your kidneys, which makes hormones to control your blood pressure, drugs to control blood pressure are almost always needed. This is the one area I am still working on to correct. But I think it may take some artificial means of reversing the DNA or gene damage that causes this high blood pressure in the first place.

The best thing I found to help my kidneys was a concentrated Chinese herbal product called Kidney Well. I always use Kidney Well and Alisma together. But you can get products from the same company for whatever your chronic kidney disease is. Visit their web site at http://www.getwellnatural.com for their great kidney products. I use Kidney Well as often as I can; which is at least every 2-3 months. It always helps. I usually take anywhere from 6-10 tablets of Kidney Well and 2-3 capsules of Alisma per dose 3 times daily on an empty stomach. It's good to take one of those doses right before bed time. There are no side effects to this herbal remedy, except maybe for some light stomach pains or discomfort occasionally. It gives you a clean feeling.

When it comes to holding down your protein, I have found that red meat is the hardest on your kidneys. So it was easy for me to get off red meat and just eat Omega-3 rich fish, and chicken and turkey. You should take Bromelain with meals that include meat. Bromelain breaks down protein real well and is a natural product made from pineapple. Bromelain is also good at flushing excess protein out of your kidneys; a common problem for those with chronic kidney disease. Using Bromelain and papaya enzyme helps take the load off your pancreas in its role in digestion; which helps prevent diabetes.

Be sure to follow the instructions to cure Diabetes, since Diabetes is the cause of 90% of kidney patients reaching end stage renal failure.

I drank gallons of Goji, Noni and Mangosteen Juice and ate Goji berries over the time since first being diagnosed with chronic kidney disease. Regardless of any rumors of these being miracle cures, the extremely high anti-oxidant properties was reason enough to use these juices and berries. The problem is finding the rare few pure juices. (See more in the next chapter under Goji, Noni and Mangosteen.)

Stop cooking with the microwave. Only use the microwave to heat things for 30 seconds or less. The damage cooking in a microwave does to food turns a good meal into a bad meal for your health. Microwaving food destroys up to 97% of the delicate vitamins and phytonutrients, plant medicines, in food.

If your doctor tries to trick you with white lies about your PTH hormone levels being high and you are on a CCB, Calcium channel blocker, like Amlodipine, then ask your doctor to take you off the calcium channel blocker and switch it to an ACE inhibitor such as Quinapril, aka Accupril. Your Parathyroid glands control calcium levels in your body. Once your Parathyroid glands sense that the calcium channel blocker is blocking calcium to your heart, your Parathyroid glands will begin to release hormones, PTH. This causes your system to start releasing calcium from your bones into your blood stream to make up for that "simulated" calcium deficiency. Doctors only want you to do another drug to control the side effects of the first drug, the calcium channel blocker.

Avoid taking Ibuprofen, naproxen and aspirin. All of these are hard on your kidneys. Follow the instructions for **Headaches** to avoid the need for any of these over the counter drugs. Tylenol is hard on your liver. I have only taken a few Aleve in the past 5 years, and that was for severe tooth or back pain.

Your big problem is usually controlling your Potassium. Potassium is in just about everything you eat, but is highest in beans and peas; especially green beans. So I rarely eat any beans or peas. An 8-ounce serving of beans has as much Potassium as 3 or 4 oranges or bananas. I never eat more than 2 oranges or bananas in a day. One of each is as far as I go. Cutting down on meat portions will help limit protein and Potassium too. Eating cheese and drinking milk and orange juice should be held to a minimum if you want to control your Potassium. Eight ounces of milk or orange juice contains around 300mg of Potassium which is the same amount of Potassium in one medium orange or banana. One thing I have noticed is that even when I eat Potassium rich fruits, it doesn't seem to have the Potassium raising effect that meats have.

So lean toward eating fresh fruits and vegetables. I wish we could get watermelon year round. I am always thrilled to eat good watermelon. It is nothing but good for you. It is a great source of distilled water. A funny thing that is true is that if you really want the best detox program for your body, eat watermelon and soak in a hot tub as much as you can. Cantaloupe is great for the same reasons. You will notice how you have to pee more often after eating either one too.

There aren't really any vitamins I take just for the kidneys. But I do take vitamins and herbs that do help my kidneys such as fish and flax seed oil, Taurine, Vitamin C, Vitamin E, B-Complex, L-Arginine, Astragalus and Bilberry. And the Kidney Well is a formula of about 5 herbs which includes Astragalus and Alisma. But make sure you steer clear of herbs like Licorice Root and Celery Seed. You can take Celery Seed as a diuretic as long as you are sure that your kidneys are not inflamed. Taking amino acids, B-Complex, will provide a lot of those B Vitamins you'll lose by restricting your protein consumption.

You can read Dr. Mackenzie Walser's book titled Coping With Kidney Disease: A 12-Step Program to Avoid Dialysis. His book gives you detailed information and instructions on restricting your protein intake. He kept lots of people off dialysis for years by putting his patients on protein restricted diets. He was a doctor and professor at the well-known John Hopkins Medical Center and University. His book was the only help I got from a doctor before I met Dr. Moskowitz.

As long as your creatinine isn't above 3.9, Dr. Moskowitz can probably keep you off dialysis. And even if your creatinine is 3.9 or above, he is still willing to help you. Between his treatment and what I did to help my kidneys, as told in this book, I do not know of a single other thing that can help anyone with chronic kidney disease. But hey, the entire medical profession can't and does not do a thing to help the kidneys of chronic kidney disease patients. They only treat the symptoms of CKD while they hold your hand and lead you to the dialysis machine and the grave.

Kidney stones – Kidney stones are cured the same way bladder stones and bone spurs are cured. So, also read the cures for bladder stones and bone spurs. The one factor that makes kidney stones different is the effect of uric acid in forming kidney stones. Over production of Uric acid is what causes gout. But its role in forming kidney stones is what separates kidney stones from bladder stones and bone spurs.

Too much Uric acid for prolonged periods of time leads to uric acid stones. Uric acid is produced when purines break up. Purines are found in foods like peas, beans, liver and some alcoholic drinks. So avoid a diet high in animal protein. It is very important to drink a lot of water to help prevent and cure kidney stones. You can't allow excess uric crystals to remain in the kidneys and form these uric acid stones. Drinking 2-3 quarts of pure water a day will help pass around 90% of kidney stones. So don't forget!

And don't forget the magnesium, if you have calcium kidney stones, which will dissolve this most common type of kidney stones. B6 also acts like Magnesium in the body. And read the cure for bladder stones.

To cure calcium based kidney stones, you do the same things you do to cure bladder stones and bone spurs – take plenty of magnesium. But to cure Uric acid stones, you need to drink baking soda water. This will dissolve Uric acid stones, much like the way Magnesium will prevent and dissolve calcium based kidney stones to cure you. Drinking plenty of water helps flush these stones out.

Make sure you read the complete information about curing kidney stones in chapter 11 in What If My Kidney Problem is Kidney stones?

Leg cramps - If it's just cramps, you need salt; preferably sea salt or eat pretzels and tomato juice. But if your calves tighten up real hard, it's lack of Potassium. I had the intense tightening of my calves just before my kidneys went out. I had to run to the bathtub and run hot water on my calves to help. If these vise grip leg cramps happen very often, you should have the doctor do a BMP or CMP to check kidney function. Your kidneys control the levels of nutrients in your blood. So lack of Potassium would be caused by your kidneys. You can increase your Potassium levels by eating bananas, oranges, peas, beans and Orange Juice NOT FROM CONCENTRATE. Or take chelated Potassium. This should correct the problem in about 3-6 weeks unless your kidneys are bad or your problem is lack of salt.

A trick I learned was to take 600mg Alpha Lipoic Acid for 4-6 weeks. This causes your kidneys to reuse Potassium and other nutrients. So it's like doubling or tripling your Potassium without a diet adjustment. It's best to get the CMP or BMP in case your kidneys are going bad.

And wear socks to bed to keep your calves warm. Also, read this simple link http://answers.google.com/answers/threadview/id/707090.html. The socks will help, but won't solve the problem. It might also be dehydration. Drink 1-ounce of water for every 2 pounds body weight. But chlorine and fluoride in the water is bad for you. So drink less unless you have a water filter. My leg cramps for years were like vise grips and by far the worst cramps of my life. I suffered for years until I learned what I told you here. I have never had them the past few years since I solved the problem. Also, stretching your muscles all over your body helps relieve lots of old age body aches. Taking Fish oil daily helps too. So does magnesium, since Magnesium helps relax muscles, including your heart.

Liver Disease – Every case of liver disease is caused by some kind of a chemical. The only exceptions are the ones caused by a virus. Actually, Hepatitis is the actual cause of those cases of liver disease. But Hepatitis is caused by a virus; although some cases of Hepatitis are caused by poisons. This comes from the Medical profession, such as the Mayo Clinic. The list of chemicals known to cause liver disease is pretty long. It includes over the counter pain relievers such as aspirin, acetaminophen, ibuprofen or naproxen.

Most of us already know that alcohol causes liver disease. Well, actually it's excess alcohol over a period of time that does. But even your birth control pills can cause liver disease. Even excess use of specific herbs such as Kava, Black Cohosh and Valerian Root can cause liver disease; as well as chemical herbicides, insecticides and pesticides.

The overall common factor is repeated consumption or exposure to these substances. Some you have complete control over. Others you need help to identify and avoid. That's why I wrote this book. Your body is great at ridding itself of these chemicals and poisons. But the precise problem is how we all accept our food, drinks, water and just about everything being full of poisons, as safe. No one really thinks about this. This is what you are doing and you know it. So take a long look at the poisons you have complete control over and begin to limit or do without them altogether - the over the counter medicines, birth control pills and yard, home and garden chemicals you are using.

And work on cutting down on the alcohol. You should hold it to 2 ounces of alcohol a day. But at least work on drinking less. Alcohol affects the mind and therefore your behavior. So trying to talk you into drinking less or stop is not ever going to work. It's your life and health. All me or anyone can do is give you the help you need to change things. But it is YOU that has to do it for yourself. Science is against you having a positive outcome when you drink excessively.

Your liver will become diseased by overloading it with hard poisons like those mentioned above. This is the truth about your kidneys too. They are the two organs that rid your body of all poisons and body metabolism waste and excesses. **Your liver can regenerate new liver cells and replace lost mass. That is, if you have part of your liver removed, it will grow back.** An herb known to accelerate liver cell regeneration is Milk Thistle. This liver cell regeneration is pronounced in those with alcohol induced cirrhosis of the liver.

Milk Thistle contains a bioflavonoid complex known as silymarin. Milk Thistle accelerates liver cell regeneration by reinforcing protein synthesis in liver cells. It is a powerful antioxidant which protects liver cells by blocking toxins from entering the liver and removing them. Milk Thistle has been used by Europeans for thousands of years as an herbal treatment for liver disorders. There are other herbs you may want to consider to help your liver disease, such as chicory seed, caper bush and yarrow. You can research these particular herbs to see if they would be good for your liver disease. I have used all of these herbs as part of a preventative for liver disease.

Excess sugar consumption causes your liver to convert the glucose and fructose in sugar to a lipid, fat. The liver quickly converts fructose in sugar and HFCS to fat molecules called triglycerides. This is what clogs your arteries and causes high blood pressure. **Choline is a B vitamin that's required for the transport of fat out of the liver.** Using Choline supplements will work fine. Some good sources of Choline in foods are Beef liver, eggs, Ground Beef, Cauliflower, Navy Beans, Almonds, Peanut Butter and Tofu.

Choline also protects the liver from certain types of damage and can help to reverse damage that has already occurred. Choline protects our liver from fat accumulating in our liver. So those with any type of liver disease should make a habit of taking Choline.

And remember to drink lots of pure water. You need lots of water to help your kidneys and liver flush those disease causing toxins out of your body. Taking as many anti-oxidants as you can will speed along the removal of those toxins. Taking immune boosting herbs like Astragalus will boost this process too and speed your healing. But recognizing and avoiding poisons has to always be your main concern in curing and preventing liver disease. So make sure you have read the chapters about poisons in your food, drinks and water to guide you in doing so.

Increasing circulation to the liver by exercising the abdominal muscles will help improve your liver, as well as any aerobic exercise or yoga.

Menopause symptoms – For menopause symptoms you need to take Black Cohosh, Eleuthero (Siberian Ginseng), Calcium D-Glucarate, Zinc, Iron and calcium. Valerian Root is good for cramps, but use it with caution at the minimum dose. Black Cohosh helps balance hormones and prevent or limit hot flashes. Eleuthero boosts your immune system and your concentration, as well as relieves stress. Zinc is essential for reproductive organs, while iron is for blood health to avoid anemia. Iron is an essential part of blood hemoglobin.

Valerian root is a natural sedative and calms the nerves and helps cramps. A better alternative is drinking Chamomile tea. Chamomile was one of the Egyptians' cure alls, but is best known to promote calm and relieve anxiety.

Sinus pressure – To relieve sinus pressure take Bee Propolis. My wife has had some sinus problems and tried a lot of things. She found out on her own that Bee Propolis was supposed to help with sinus conditions. We had some around for years for other reasons, but my wife had never tried it. When all else failed, she tried the Bee Propolis to see if it would help. Sure enough, the Bee Propolis caused all that yellowish snotty stuff in her sinuses to come out within a few hours and relief came with that. Since then, others have tried the same thing and said it was almost like a miracle how it cleaned out their sinuses. My wife still has some sinus problems on occasion, but she takes care of it with the Bee Propolis. So it's always short lived.

Another way to relieve sinus pressure is to flush your sinuses with a saline solution made of 4 ounces warm water, ¼ teaspoon salt and 1/8 teaspoon baking soda. Flush your sinuses with this solution using something like a bulb syringe. We got one with our ear wax flush. Use these natural methods to try and rid yourself of the drugs you usually use for these conditions.

Stress – Stress affects everyone. But few people know how to deal with stress or even begin to. Dealing with most stress is really quite easy. Dealing with all your stress takes a bit more effort and time. To deal with most stress, obvious stress, here is what you do. Simply say the word "Relax" in your head and repeat it slower and more softly as you repeat the word "Relax". It's best to sit while you do this, but it also works standing up or laying down. Your muscles are already tense just to keep you standing up. Once you've said "Relax" a few times, start saying "I refuse to be tense" a few times. Then alternate between the two phrases slower and softer as you repeat those two phrases. This also helps you to recognize other places in your body that are tense.

As you recognize those new places, continue doing the same thing, alternately saying those two phrases – Relax and I refuse to be tense. And add "I resist all tension" right after you say "I refuse to be tense" each time. So you start out with just relax, then work in "I refuse to be tense". Then add the phrase "I resist all tension". The reason this works so well is because your body develops tension through natural activities. You have to interrupt your body and mind and dwell on the opposite. Relax is the opposite of tension. So you tell your body to relax AND to resist that tension and resist ALL that tension. It's best to breathe deeply through your nose and exhale through your mouth, after holding it for a few seconds while you do all of this.

Almost all stress raises your blood pressure. And once you pile one source of tension on top of another and another, you are adversely affecting your health. I got rid of all my stress several years ago, and have managed to stay rid of almost all stress. It took some work. But I did it. If my pets do something to piss me off, I just refuse to be mad, relax and let it go. Then deal with the mess the pet made. It's so easy to rear up and get mad. We all do in those situations. But your health is far more important than you getting rightfully angry.

Someone can insult you or call you names, and you CAN get pissed off. But is your health really worth sacrificing just to get pissed off at being called names or insult. Damn! You've already been insulted and called names. And now you're going to intentionally get stressed out and get that blood pressure up!

Treat yourself better than that and don't get pissed off. Relax and resist that tension and anger. Do that for yourself! Being angry does have bad effects on the health of your body and mind; especially your heart and circulatory system.

Strokes – Strokes are caused by the same things that cause heart attacks. Both are caused by blood clots or blood vessels bursting for the most part. So do the same things for Strokes as outlined under **Heart Disease.** And also read the cure for Alzheimer's disease, since it explains things you can do to achieve good brain health.

Tennis Elbow – Tendinitis – Buy this book and do what he shows you to do to cure your tennis elbow – http://www.tenniselbowtips.com. This worked for my wife. It's some simple low impact exercises to strengthen your tendons to cure you, using things like rubber bands, a can of food, a hammer and such.

Underarm lumps (knots) – Those knots, lumps, under your arms are caused by the aluminum compounds in your underarm deodorants. Aluminium chloride, aluminium chlorohydrate, and aluminium-zirconium compounds and most notably aluminum zirconium tetrachlorohydrex gly and aluminum zirconium trichlorohydrex gly are frequently used in antiperspirants. Aluminium chlorohydrate and aluminium zirconium tetrachlorohydrate gly are the most frequent active ingredients in commercial antiperspirants. So if you have lumps or knots in your arm pits, then stop using that deodorant with an aluminum based ingredient. It's that simple.

I had lumpy hard knots on my arm pits for a decade or more. I stopped using the aluminum based deodorants I was using and the knots went away in about 3 weeks. I went without deodorant most of that time, because I couldn't find a deodorant that did NOT have aluminum in it. I finally found some Old Spice that only had glycol in it. It doesn't plug your underarm sweat ducts like the aluminum ones do. But I healed myself of those knots and haven't had any lumps since the first half of 2007.

What makes this type of poisoning so bad is that your lymph glands are right there beneath your underarms. So you are sending poisons almost directly to your lymph glands, which is part of your immunes system.

Varicose veins – Take Butcher's Broom for varicose veins. Doing so will flatten your varicose veins and fortify your vessel wall muscles. Butcher's Broom is also known to relieve the itching, swelling and burning in your legs. 400mg daily is a good dose. Wrapping cold towels around your varicose veins can also help.

A few last words about cures and preventions.................

No matter what the disease is, it's almost always going to be caused by toxins. The problem is how we are blind to these poisons. Just because the FDA certifies them "safe" doesn't make them safe. You have to learn what these poisons are and read the labels to avoid as many poisons as you can. In this country, there isn't a way for any of us to avoid poisons in our food and drinks. But you sure can filter out 99% of the poisons in your water with a fluoride water filter or better. And that is the first thing you need to do, so you can start drinking 1-ounce of water for every 2 pounds of body weight daily.

Then get off that red meat, or at least cut back on it. Try sticking with just ground chuck. Eat fish as often as possible. Eat Cod, Salmon, Tuna, Tilapia and other cold water fish that have scales. Catfish is NOT one of them. Eat as many fresh fruits and vegetables as you can. I mean FRESH! Cooking produce kills the life-giving enzymes in live food. So buy produce you can eat raw first. Then buy frozen vegetables and fruits as your second choice. And cook those fruits and vegetables only if you must! Buy canned only as a last resort.

I know that some of the diseases and medical conditions didn't have a decisive cure. But the principles I learned trying to save my own life turned out to cure every disease and medical condition I had. Sure you like to swig down soda pops and fruit juices. But is Diabetes, Kidney disease, headaches, heartburn, internal bleeding and all the rest worth blindly scarfing down all these poisons? You have indulged and over indulged long enough.

Now put these food and drink vices aside and use them in moderation only, so your body can spend its energy repairing cells in your body to make you well. And add the things your body is lacking, starting with Magnesium and Omega-3. Take these, Vitamin C and the other lesser known of the antioxidants, like Selenium, Alpha Lipoic Acid and Vitamins E and A.

I can never quite express just how shocked I was to cure myself of all the things I did. I only wanted to help my kidneys; since my kidneys proved they were soaked with poisons. Doing liver, kidney, candida, colon and other cleanses and detoxification aids certainly helps to get the poisons OUT, once you put them IN your body. But **you can certainly agree that not putting those poisons in your body in the first place is a far better and more cost efficient way of dealing with all those poisons.** Once inside, these poisons do their damage. And it could all be avoided by never putting those poisons in your body in the first place. You just have to know what the poisons are so you can look for them and avoid them.

I hope you are saying "I read that in your book already many times." If so, I can only say "GREAT!!!!". Hey, once you know what causes something, you eliminate that cause as the main part of the solution to that problem. Once you do that, then you need to know how to repair the damage. That is what this chapter is about. It's about the things you need to be doing FOR your body, now that the cause of that problem has been eliminated.

You can clean up your car and make it shine. But unless you put gas in the tank, it's not gonna run at all. And it sure won't run on bad fuel or junk! So get rid of those poisons, like most of this book dwells on. And give your body the things it needs to nourish itself and stay healthy.

You can cure yourself while you still keep the same relationship you've always had with your doctors. If you follow the advice in this book, the difference will be that now you've added cures to your life. And those cures cost a fraction of what the treatments do! It's your body and your life. You are the one that is with YOU 24 hours a day. You could be helping yourself all the time. You only see a doctor for an hour or two every once in a while! And you care about you far more than the doctors or anyone else ever could.

The information in this book empowers YOU to take control of your health and get your life back that sickness and chronic ailments have eaten away. But don't be blaming me or claiming I'm a liar when you get heartburn after eating 5 honey buns and some chocolate milk or after drinking a big Super-sized drink and some Oreos. Don't bad mouth ME because you chugged down all those beers and ate a platter of shrimp and got gout! Or you keep on drinking alcohol and smoking cigarettes habitually and have one stroke after another. Get use to blaming yourself for what you do to your body. Then and only then can you start to solve the problem.

Why am I telling you this? Because I'm the idiot who made myself sick. I'm the one who did the things to give myself headaches, heartburn, arthritis, bladder stones, gout and chronic kidney disease. But hey! NOW.... I'm also the one who did the things to cure myself of one "incurable" disease after another. And I'm no better than you, as long as you have the information to do the same.

Now I will give you some more information about the Herbs, Vitamins and healing foods I have talked about.

9 - Vitamins, Herbs & Healing Foods: What Are They Used For?

This chapter is here as a companion to chapter 8 – MORE Cures and Preventions and other places in this book. You can look in chapter 8 to read specific instructions for a cure. And if you want to know more about those herbs, vitamins and healing foods mentioned in those cures and preventions, you can do so in this chapter. You can also find other diseases and medical conditions that each of these vitamins, herbs and healing foods cure, prevent or improve that are not listed in Chapter 8.

I separated the information in this chapter from the information in chapter 8, so that the specific instructions for each cure and prevention was easier for everyone to understand. Going into depth about any vitamin, herb or healing food would not remain specific to that specific disease.

For example, you don't need to know the details about Fish oil being good for arthritis in the information about gout. So I give you specific information about Fish oil and many of the things Fish oil is good for, in this chapter. Most of the information in this chapter is pretty well-known, unlike the rest of the information in this book; but not really common knowledge among the masses.

The information in this chapter is scientific facts about each of these Vitamins, Herbs and Foods. The rest of the information is from what I know by personal experience. You can find this information from many sources. I included this chapter as a convenience for those who read this book.

Also, remember to SEARCH the INTERNET for as much information as you want on any of these Vitamins, Herbs and Healing Foods.

- This printed version has these shades of gray text for – Herbs – Vitamins - and Healing Foods.

Astragalus - Astragalus is an adaptoge, meaning it helps protect the body against various stresses; including physical, mental and emotional stress. Astragalus may help protect the body from diseases such as cancer and diabetes. It contains antioxidants which protect cells against damage caused by free radicals, byproducts of cellular energy. Astragalus is used to protect and support the immune system, for preventing colds and upper respiratory infections, to lower blood pressure, to treat diabetes and to protect the liver.

Astragalus has antibacterial and anti-inflammatory properties. It is sometimes used topically for wounds. In addition, studies have shown that Astragalus has antiviral properties and stimulates the immune system; suggesting that it is indeed effective at preventing colds.

In the United States, researchers have investigated Astragalus as a possible treatment for people whose immune systems have been compromised by chemotherapy or radiation. In these studies, Astragalus supplements have been shown to speed recovery and extend life expectancy. Research on using

Astragalus for people with AIDS has produced inconclusive results.

Recent research in China indicates that Astragalus may offer antioxidant benefits to people with severe forms of heart disease; relieving symptoms and improving heart function. At low-to-moderate doses, Astragalus has few side effects, although it does interact with a number of other herbs and prescription medications. Astragalus may also have mild diuretic (rids the body of excess fluid) activity. Traditional uses include the treatment of the following:

- Anemia – Asthma - Bloating - Chronic fatigue - Colds & influenza - Diarrhea – Fatigue or lack of appetite due to chemotherapy – Fever - Heart disease - Hepatitis - Kidney disease – Multiple allergies - Persistent infection – Stomach ulcers - Stomach Gas – Stress - Wounds

Bee Propolis – Bee propolis is made by bees from tree bark and other plant materials bees collect. It is the substance bees use to protect their hives. Bee propolis contains vitamins, minerals and bioflavanoids. Bee propolis has antibacterial and anesthetic healing properties. Its fungicide and antibiotic properties date back to ancient Rome, Greece and the Egyptians. It strengthens the immune system as well. All this points to why Bee Propolis is used to combat gingivitis, bronchitis, pneumonia, sinusitis, ear infections, influenza, respiratory diseases, herpes and to treat cavities.

My wife takes Bee propolis for sinus pressure. It works better than anything to clear up her sinus pressure. After taking a couple of capsules of Bee Propolis, my wife always has a mass of yellow mucus that comes out of her nose. But she always feel so much better once it does. We both have taken Bee Propolis for sore gums; usually after getting a tooth pulled or deep cleaning at the dentist.

Bee Propolis also relieves the effects of inhaling too much dust, like when you are vacuuming without a HEPA filter or getting built off dust off your curtains, ceiling fans or similar high dust areas, even baseball fields.

Black Cohosh - The herb Black Cohosh has been used for centuries for arthritis and rheumatism as an anti-inflammatory; as well as for menstrual difficulties and for hot flashes of menopause. But women with breast cancer should avoid Black Cohosh, since Black Cohosh seems to behave like estrogen in the body. This helps since estrogen production declines during menopause. Black Cohosh also acts as a mild sedative and relieves pain after child birth. Black Cohosh is the root of a plant in the buttercup family.

Black strap Molasses – Black strap molasses (not to be confused with molasses) is a dark, sweet flavored syrup that is made by boiling sugar syrup from sugar cane or sugar beets and is mainly used as a sugar substitute. It's the third boiling of this sugar syrup that yields the black strap molasses. It is high in Potassium, calcium, copper, Magnesium and manganese; as well as iron, selenium and B6. Black strap molasses can prevent migraines, joint problems, irregular heartbeats, brain disturbances, arthritis, celiac disease, anemia and even lower your cholesterol. Some say it can even help turn your gray hair back to its original color. It's best to buy organic unsulfured black strap molasses.

Vitamin C – An antioxidant, Vitamin C prevents the free-radical damage that contributes to aging and aging-related diseases, including cancer, cardiovascular disorders and others.

A major contributor to our immune system, Vitamin C helps increase resistance to a range of diseases, including cancer. Excess Vitamin C stimulates the production of lymphocytes, an important component of our immune system. Ascorbic Acid is also required by the thymus gland, one of the major glands involved in immunity and increases the mobility of the phagocytes; the type of cell that "eats" bacteria, viral cells, and cancer cells, as well as other harmful invaders.

Vitamin C acts in many ways to help prevent high blood pressure and atherosclerosis; hardening of the arteries that can lead to heart attacks and strokes.

Vitamin C forms cementing substances such as collagen that hold body cells together, thus strengthening blood vessels. It hastens healing of wounds and bones and increases resistance to infection. Vitamin C aids in the utilization of iron, converts Folic Acid into its active form and increases our ability to absorb and store iron. It also improves the bio-availability of selenium.

Vitamin C is used by the liver to detoxify drugs and other chemicals, and appears to protect the body from the side effects that accompany many drugs.

Another important role of Vitamin C is the one it plays in our ability to handle all types of physical & mental stress.

To prevent colds, in August start taking 1000mg of Vitamin C as cold and flu season approaches. Keep this up all through the cold and flu season to prevent colds and flus. If you already have a cold or get one any way, then take 1000mg Vitamin C every 4-6 hours until you are well; usually 3-4 days later instead of 10-14 or more. Vitamin C is an essential nutrient and is also called ascorbic acid, L-ascorbic acid and L-ascorbate and should not be confused with citric acid. You will sometimes see it used in food items.

Since your body doesn't store Vitamin C, it's up to you to make sure you take Vitamin C supplements. Vitamin C is inexpensive and the most readily available anti-oxidant of all. The only natural substance I recommend in this book that is cheaper than Vitamin C is baking soda. So cost should not be a factor when choosing to take it. Vitamin C was the first vitamin to be mass produced back in 1934 when it was produced and marketed as Redoxon.

At the top of the next page is a table which shows you what dosage to take for certain diseases. This table gives a few examples to give you a good idea of how much Vitamin C you should take for those diseases and disease in general.

Here is a table for suggested Vitamin C dosage for specific conditions:

Condition	Suggested dosage in mg
allergies or asthma	3,000-7,000
bleeding gums	1,000-3,000
cancer prevention	5,000-10,000
coronary heart disease prevention	500-4,000
enhanced immunity	1,000-5,000
exposure to cigarette smoke & polluted air	1,000-5,000
high levels of stress	1,000-5,000
surgery, wounds, injuries	5,000-10,000

Calcium – Calcium is found in every cell in your body. So its importance is obvious. Calcium is used to build strong bones and teeth, where almost all the body's calcium is stored. You need a minimum of 1000mg of calcium daily. It is very important to note that calcium will cause you problems like bladder and kidney stones and bone spurs if you don't take Magnesium supplements. It takes Magnesium to dissolve the calcium to make calcium of use to your body. Without enough Magnesium to do this, calcium particles are able to bind with toxins to form bladder stones, kidney stones and bone spurs. Calcium causes your heart to contract while Magnesium causes your heart to relax; thus creating proper heart rhythm.

Calcium has been found to lower blood pressure, lower risk of colon and prostate cancer and prevents osteoporosis. You have four parathyroid glands on the back of your thyroid gland that regulate the amount of calcium in the blood and bones. Besides taking Magnesium with calcium, you should also be sure to take Vitamin D; especially during winter when you don't get much sun.

Calcium D-Glucarate – Calcium D-Glucarate is the calcium salt of D-glucaric acid, and is found naturally in the body. Since many breast cancers depend on estrogen, you should take Calcium D-Glucarate, which helps the body excrete used hormones such as estrogen. Calcium D-Glucarate is known to remove, detoxify, cancer causing carcinogens in the colon, skin, liver, breasts and lungs. Do not confuse Calcium D-Glucarate with any other form of calcium. Buy only products that state the term Calcium D-Glucarate clearly and specifically. Calcium D-Glucarate is found in many fruits and vegetables. But one 500mg tablet of Calcium D-Glucarate contains as much phytonutrient as 82 pounds of fresh fruits and vegetables.

Men may want to take Calcium D-Glucarate to help remove excess estrogen as part of your cure for erectile dysfunction. Women should take Calcium D-Glucartate to help relieve symptoms of menopause and menstrual cycles, because of its effectiveness in removing used hormones such as estrogen.

<u>Cayenne</u> – Cayenne, or cayenne pepper, is one of the most beneficial foods around. Cayenne pepper can bring amazing results for simple healing and challenging health problems. It has been scientifically proven that Cayenne pepper kills prostate cancer cells. It can stop heart attacks, help rebuild flesh harmed or destroyed by frost bite, heal stomach ulcers, rebuild stomach tissue and heal hemorrhoids. In your circulatory system, cayenne improves blood circulation, rebuilds blood cells, lowers cholesterol, emulsifies triglycerides, removes toxins from the blood stream and improves the overall health of your heart, as well your blood pressure.

Cayenne can also heal your gall bladder and remove plaque from your artery walls. It has also been known to be an effective diuretic and help in both urine elimination and built up fecal matter in the intestines like colon cleansing products do. There is so much to say about cayenne peppers. The reason you don't hear about this powerful healing medicine is that the medical profession is in the business of making money, not healing people. If they were, cayenne pepper would be at the top of their list. But they haven't even mentioned it yet!

Taking Cayenne and Garlic has been known to cure stomach ulcers too. You would think it would make it worse. But that is just not the truth.

<u>Chromium GTF</u> – Chromium GTF is a niacin bound absorbable form of the mineral chromium and is named for the way it interacts with insulin. Chromium deficiency hampers insulin function and energy levels. So if you are a diabetic, chromium GTF can be a huge plus for your health. Chromium GTF improves your blood lipid profiles such as LDL cholesterol and triglycerides; which lowers your blood pressure. 400mcg is a proper daily dose for adults.

<u>Vitamin D</u> – Vitamin D is a fat soluble vitamin that helps build strong bones, and regulate the immune system and cells. Your body stores Vitamin D and also makes it when your skin is exposed to sunlight. There are two kinds of Vitamin D - Vitamin D2 (ergocalciferol) and Vitamin D3 (cholecalciferol) which is the preferred form. It has been known to help prevent Diabetes, SAD, heart disease, obesity and even Multiple Sclerosis. You should take around 400IU of Vitamin D daily; preferably in two doses.

<u>Vitamin E</u> – Vitamin E is a fat soluble vitamin that comes in two forms. The natural form is d-alpha tocopherol while the synthetic form is dl-alpha tocopherol. It is an antioxidant that is known to thin the blood, prevent cholesterol from oxidizing and clinging to blood vessels, helps repair damaged cells, protects cell membranes and promotes cell growth. Vitamin E does a near miraculous job of healing burns, cuts and other wounds to the skin. I call it an internal and external healer. If you apply Vitamin E to a cut, or stitched wound, the Vitamin E will heal the wound so well that you will barely be able to tell you

were ever cut. It has the same healing power inside the body too. Vitamin E is one of the most useful antioxidants for these reasons. I even use Vitamin E on my pets to heal their cuts or damaged skin. Signs of Vitamin E deficiency are weak muscles and fertility problems. So Vitamin E is a preventive for both. A dose of 400IU daily will work as a preventive.

But if you are already sick or wounded, you can take as much as 1500IU daily for a short period of time, 3-6 weeks most days. As with any Vitamin, try to take the total amount in 2 or more doses each day. Those who take the drug Warfarin should be cautioned about the risk of increased bleeding possible with a dose of Vitamin E higher than 400IU daily.

Fish oil - Fish oil and Omega-3 are known to have many health benefits. As a matter of fact, I have mentioned Fish oil many times in this book because the so-called American diet is so deficient in Omega-3. Almost every person in this country suffers the effects of not being on a fish diet as man is supposed to be. Fish oils contain the Omega-3 fatty acids eicosapentaenoic acid (EPA) and docosahexaenoic acid (DHA); precursors of eicosanoids that are known to reduce inflammation throughout the body. Fish oil comes from the tissues of oily fish such as cod, haddock, salmon, trout, sardine, herring and mackerel. Fish oil is high in Vitamins A and D and Omega-3 fatty acids. Its most well-known benefits are in helping those with heart disease, depression and inflammatory conditions such as arthritis. Fish oil is an anti-inflammatory.

Some of the conditions that Fish oil cures, prevents or improves are depression, peptic ulcers, Alzheimer's disease, Chron's disease, Colitis, Breast Cancer, lupus and heart disease. Fish oil also improves your skin, promotes weight loss, prevents schizophrenia, eases bi-polar disorders, improves brain function, increases eye focus and much more. The EFAs, essential fatty acids, in Fish oil fight the plaque in the brain that causes Alzheimer's. Those already afflicted with Alzheimer's disease can reduce the symptoms of Alzheimer's.

Fish oil emulsifies the plaque that clings to your artery and blood vessel walls which causes high blood pressure, hardening of the arteries, heart attacks and strokes. It acts like a scavenger to clean your blood and make your blood flow more smoothly. It also cures arthritis by lubricating the joints and acting as an anti-inflammatory to reduce the pain and swelling associated with arthritis. Fish oil is also beneficial to the pancreas and strengthens a weak pancreas. It is also a strong ally against cancer of the pancreas.

Fish oil is proven to prevent and cure breast cancer. It kills breast cancer cells as fast as chemotherapy. This is because of the high fat content in women's breasts; which almost every woman is seriously deficient in, due to not being on a fish diet.

Out of all the deficiencies in your diet, the lack of Omega-3 is the most problematic of all deficiencies, followed by Magnesium. That is why I advise every one to take Fish oil and Magnesium as their first items to take; after you get that water filter for your kitchen and shower. I take Fish oil, flax seed oil and other oils containing EFAs like Primrose oil and Extra Virgin Olive oil. Primrose oil contains GLA; which is the most biologically active form of Omega-6 fatty acid. Other oils with good sources of Omega-3 are squid, krill, algal and hemp.

You can get good quality Fish oil at Puritan's Pride. The Fish oil we buy is found at **www.puritan.com/nutritional-oils-068/omega-3-fish-oil-1200-mg-013326**.

If you have any chronic disease or condition, take 3000-5000mg Fish oil daily for 3-6 weeks, then back off to a maintenance dose of 1000-1200mg daily or most days. If this does not cure a disease or condition known to be cured by Fish oil, then take the larger dose several weeks longer.

And make sure you do your own research to find out all the different diseases and medical conditions that Fish oil helps. There's so much more to learn than what I have included in this book. But merely taking Fish oil as an all-around preventative is one of the very smartest things you can do for your health.

Flax seed – Flax seed is the vegetable form of Omega-3; whereas Fish oil is the animal form. Flax seed oil can be used in place of Fish oil, but the combination of the two seem to provide the greatest benefits. The same things said about Fish oil above, are also true about flax seed and flax seed oil; though flax seed oil is the most beneficial in preventing and curing breast cancer. So make sure you read back over the information on Fish oil when using flax seed.

Garlic – Garlic is one of the most potent natural medicines of all time. It contains over 400 health enhancing chemical compounds; making it an all-natural medicinal treasure chest. The most powerful compound from garlic is allicin. Allicin is produced when garlic is chopped or crushed. So the more crushing or chopping, the more allicin is generated; thus increasing the medicinal effect. Allicin has an excellent antibiotic, anti-fungal ability. Powerful sulfur compounds in garlic kill and inhibit an amazing array of fungi, viruses, molds, bacteria and even worms and parasites.

Among the things garlic can do is lower cholesterol and blood sugar, detoxifies, strengthens the immune system, inhibits cancer, treats HIV/AIDS infections, fights respiratory diseases, lowers blood pressure as well as killing herpes on contact.

Garlic has been known for its healing powers for several thousand years. It's best to eat garlic raw; crushed or chopped. But a lot of people prefer to take garlic oil capsules. Dry garlic tablets are the least desirable. Take 1000mg daily as a preventative and 3000-5000mg for 3-6 weeks if you have a disease or condition which garlic is known to cure or help.

I haven't ever heard of anyone having adverse effects from garlic, except for having occasional "garlic breath". Garlic needs to stay high on your list of healing foods along with Fish oil. The Garlic we buy at Puritan's Pride is at **http://www.puritan.com/garlic-060/garlic-oil-1000-mg-002970?NewPage=1#product**.

Goji – Goji berries and juice are valued for their nutrient and antioxidant value and content. The ORAC value for rating antioxidant value of foods is at least six times that of any other fruit or berry you can buy in the grocery store. Goji is also known as the Wolfberry, which grows mainly in China in the Himalayas. The problem you run into with buying Goji is how juice manufacturers only offer Goji juice mixed with cheaper fruit juices to try and fool customers into paying high prices for their products labeled "Goji Juice". So you have to find the rare few that are pure Goji Juice and say so in the ingredients. You need to buy Goji juice from a place like **Healing Noni** or **Ebay**.

The best place that I have found to buy Goji and Noni juice is from Healing Noni at http://www.healingnoni.com/catalog/-c-10.html. I resorted to buying dry Goji berries after I got tired of being ripped off by one product after another with their misleading labels to trick you into buying their bottles of diluted Goji juice. I want the health benefits of Goji, not pear juice, apple juice and the other juices they use to dilute high potency healing juices like Noni and Mangosteen.

I even have several Goji Berry bushes in my yard. I've only had them 3 or 4 years. So they haven't started producing many berries yet. I like to take the dry berries and soak them in a cup of water so that I can eat them. They have an unusual taste, but not a bad taste at all. Most people would like the taste. The same is true about the pure juices.

Drink 2-4 ounces of pure juice a day and/or eat 2-4 ounces of berries or more. Goji berries and juice will be a big boost to your health if you use it. Don't fall for the gimmick advertising about Goji being a miracle healer. But never underestimate its superior nutrient and high antioxidant value.

Hawthorn Berries – Hawthorn Berry is known for its effectiveness in promoting the health of the circulatory system and treating congestive heart failure, angina, cardiac arrhythmia, chest pain and high blood pressure. Hawthorn Berry acts as a vasodilator to lower blood pressure. It also helps reduce the production of cholesterol in your liver and prevents plaque formation. Hawthorn Berry is widely regarded as safe. It is also used to treat insomnia and diarrhea. It also strengthens blood vessels, helps prevent blood clots, builds the heart muscle wall, as well as being an excellent aid in digestion.

Honey – Use only raw honey. It's cloudy, unlike worthless honey which is clear brown, like the Honey Bear brand. Real honey comes from local bee farms. We buy ours that way. Raw honey contains valuable live enzymes, vitamins and pollen that is missing from processed honey. Raw honey can be used on wounds externally and has a whole host of benefits inside the body. Some of those include the treatment of liver and kidney disorders, colds, insomnia, bad complexions, a weak heart, constipation and arthritic conditions.

Honey enters the bloodstream rapidly to give you quick energy because it is a pre-digested food which speeds up the burning of fat and stimulates the heart. It also improves your immune system by making your digestive system healthier. Raw honey also cures and prevents Botulism. Using raw honey with cinnamon also has some impressive benefits.

These benefits include aid for Arthritis, Bladder infections, Cholesterol, Colds, upset stomach, indigestion (gas), immune system, influenza, pimples, weight loss, skin infections, bad breath, cancer, fatigue and even hearing loss. Taking equal parts of honey and cinnamon powder twice daily restores hearing.

Lemon Balm – Lemon Balm is a perennial herb in the mint family. Lemon balm, along with chamomile, were used as cure alls by ancient Egyptians. The health benefits of lemon balm include improvement of digestion and memory. Lemon balm leaves are abundant in certain chemicals, such as protocatechuic, rosmarinic and caffeic acid, flavonoids and phenolic compounds, which in turn contribute to the various health benefits.

Research has confirmed the antioxidant activity of lemon balm extract. It also decreases the risk of cancer. Lemon Balm, Melissa officinalis, plays a vital role in the treatment of hyperactivity, a common disorder in children. Distraction, hyperactivity and impulsiveness are the three common features of the Attention Deficit Hyperactivity Disorder (ADHD). A significant improvement in the memory performance and cognitive functioning can occur with supplementation of dried lemon balm leaf.

Certain individuals with dyspepsia are seen to improve with a supplement of lemon balm, in combination with peppermint, licorice root, caraway and candy tuft. Leaves of lemon balm can play an important role in the treatment of flu, lowering of blood pressure, improving memory, releasing of certain hormones, treatment of depression and thyroid and relief of insomnia or sleeplessness. Lemon balm tea is useful for thyroid problems.

Grave's disease is a condition associated with the excessive production of the thyroid hormone. It is an autoimmune disorder and lemon balm decreases the secretion of the thyroid hormone. Lemon balm is also used as a nerve tonic. It also relaxes the muscles of the bladder, stomach and uterus.

This may explain what I was feeling when I drank lemon balm tea the week my kidneys blew out and I was pissing blood and blood clots. The lemon balm tea went down my throat and immediately began giving me a warm relaxed feeling in my throat which spread and flowed to my stomach and intestines. I stopped pissing blood after drinking lemon balm tea. I just figured it was proving itself as the cure all Egyptians believed it is.

Lemon balm is also good at relieving headaches and is effective against herpes simplex, dementia, Alzheimer's disease, lip sores and spasms. Its antiseptic properties make it good for treating allergies, acne and skin rashes.

Lemon balm is also good for keeping insects and flies away and out of your house. Just clean your kitchen and toilet seats with an infusion of lemon balm to keep the bugs away. And of course, you can use lemon balm to add lemon flavor to any dish like fish or barbecued meat and chicken. Lemon balm goes well with allspice, mint, pepper, rosemary and thyme.

Magnesium – Magnesium dissolves calcium to make it available for use by the body. Lack of Magnesium leaves particles of calcium available to combine with free radicals to form bladder and kidney stones and bone spurs. Magnesium also relaxes the heart to maintain proper heart rhythm, helps regulate blood sugar levels, promotes normal blood pressure, maintains normal muscle and nerve function and keeps bones strong.

Magnesium is needed for over 300 body metabolisms and is the fourth most abundant mineral in your body. About half that amount is found in your bones. Magnesium seems to be very good at helping to prevent or improve such diseases as diabetes, hypertension and cardiovascular disease.

Magnesium can also relieve migraines and tension headaches, as well as PMS discomforts like bloating, tender breasts and swelling of your upper body.

Since our food supply is so low in Magnesium because of all the processed food items that dominate it, I highly recommend you take Magnesium oxide supplements. Take 400mg daily or most days as a maintenance/preventative dose. Take at least twice that daily if you have any disease or medical condition which Magnesium is known to cure or improve.

I would tell you Magnesium can work miracles, but I would be lying. Oh wait! I have to say Magnesium can cure you of bladder stones in just a few minutes, because that was my experience. I don't want to guarantee you will get the same immediate results. But I certainly did. Just 45 minutes after taking 2 400mg Magnesium oxide tablets my fourth bladder stone attack stopped and I never had another one since then; which was 1996. It's that same thing I have told you several times already - that calcium is dissolved by magnesium, so that calcium is of use to your body. Excess doses of Magnesium will dissolve small bladder and kidney stones and bone spurs.

You need to take both Fish oil and magnesium; since these supply the two substances that most everyone in this country is deficient in.

Mangosteen – Mangosteen is a slow growing tropical evergreen tree that grows anywhere from 20 to 80 feet tall. It is native to Southeast Asia, but can also grow in places like Californian and Florida where they have year round warm humid climates. Mangosteen contains a naturally occurring poly phenolic compound called xanthones. Xanthones are anti-oxidants being researched for their ability to improve immune systems and have anti-viral, anti-bacterial, and anti-fungal properties. Xanthones and their derivatives have been shown to have several benefits, including anti-inflammatory properties, anti-allergic and anti convulsant abilities.

There are also other components of the Mangosteen that have medicinal qualities, including polysaccharides, sterols, proanthocyanidins and catechins. These are less nutritionally important and biologically active than xanthones. But they are still a major part of what gives the fruit its medicinal benefits, since many of them act as antioxidants.

One of the most important health benefits of Mangosteen is its effect on the cardiovascular system. It is believed to be effective in preventing diseases like arthritis, cataracts, osteoporosis, high blood pressure, atherosclerosis, kidney stones, glaucoma, Alzheimer's, neuralgia, and more. It is also said that this fruit can be effective in treating depression, aging, obesity, skin diseases, allergies, ulcers, diarrhea, fevers and pain.

But just as it is with Goji juice, you have to be aware that 99% of what is sold as Mangosteen juice barely has any Mangosteen in it. The best I have found is Adam's Mangosteen juice at www.mangosteens.com. It's the only Mangosteen juice I care to buy any more. Adam's is far better than advertised Mangosteen juices such as Xango and MangoXan. Adam's is 100% Mangosteen juice. Each bottle has over 10 pounds of Mangosteen. I usually drink about 4 ounces a day when I have any Mangosteen juice. You shouldn't expect Mangosteen to be a miracle cure or replace good nutrition. The "miracle cures" come from eliminating poisons and correcting specific nutrition deficiencies.

Niacin - Niacin is a type of B vitamin. It is water-soluble, which means it is not stored in the body. Water-soluble vitamins dissolve in water. Leftover amounts of the vitamin leave the body through the urine. That means you need a continuous supply of such vitamins in your diet. Niacin is also known as Nicotinic acid and Vitamin B3. Niacin assists in the functioning of the digestive system, skin, and nerves. It is also important for the conversion of food to energy. Niacin acts as an important co-factor needed for the proper functioning of over 50 enzymes. Enzymes are proteins needed for all the chemical reactions that make life possible.

Live fresh produce is a great source of enzymes. But once you cook or freeze the produce, you kill the enzymes. Killing the enzymes is why you have to cook most produce before you can or freeze them for storage.

No vitamin, hormone, or mineral can exert its beneficial effects in the body without the help of enzymes. Niacin helps the body produce energy and metabolize fat and cholesterol and helps make sex hormones and other important signal molecules. Niacin is also a structural component of Glucose Tolerance Factor (GTF) that potentiates insulin. Niacin improves its ability to bind to cell surface receptors.

Since niacin causes what is called "red flush" at doses as low as 25mg, you need to be aware of this and learn how to increase your dose of daily niacin with the least amount of discomfort. That is, unless you like the red flush! I explained how to increase your daily dose to 500mg with the least discomfort under **Heart Disease** in chapter 8.

Noni - Noni fruit and juice have been around for centuries and utilized in cultures across Southeast Asia and the South Pacific. Officially known as Morinda citrifola, Noni is a type of mulberry. It 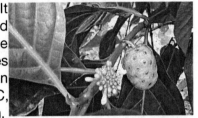 flowers year round, producing a pungent and somewhat bitter fruit and juice. The juice is the most widely used by-product, but in some cultures the leaves and roots are also used. The fruit is an excellent source of nutrients including Vitamin C, niacin, Potassium, Vitamin A, calcium and sodium.

Research has identified the presence of 10 essential vitamins, 7 dietary minerals, and 18 amino acids. Noni also contains a mixture of organic acids, anthroquinones, and xeronine.

It is xeronine that some researchers believe holds the key to Noni's potential. Noni contains significant amounts of proxeronine, a precursor to the alkaloid xeronine. An enzyme in the body helps convert proxeronine into xeronine. This effect happens most frequently when Noni is taken on an empty stomach. A University of Hawaii researcher who has studied xeronine for years believes Noni, with its proxeronine content, has potential to aid some types (although not all types) of high blood pressure, menstrual cramps, arthritis, gastric ulcers, atherosclerosis, pain relief and mental depression; among many other things. Much more study is needed to verify this and the mechanism by which it works.

Noni has been used by people with a variety of conditions. It has been used by people with immune compromising diseases like chronic fatigue syndrome to boost the immune system function. It has been reported to help stabilize blood sugar levels by diabetics and hypoglycemic. Noni has been used by individuals suffering with inflammation, joint pain, and arthritis. Some people recommend Noni to improve digestive function, remove parasites, and cleanse the digestive tract.

Similarly, others use it for ulcers, irritable bowel syndrome, constipation, and diarrhea. One study of smokers observed that total cholesterol and triglycerides improved after one month of drinking Noni juice.

There is more pure Noni juice on the market than either Goji or Mangosteen juice. But you still have to read the ingredients to make sure you are getting 100% Noni juice. We buy my Goji and Noni juice from a company called Healing Noni. To buy these, go to **http://www.healingnoni.com/catalog/** for all their juice products.

The one problem with Noni is the taste. It tastes like a weak vinegar. So you may want to mix it with Goji or Mangosteen and drink it. I can stand the taste because I know the health benefits are extremely high. I wouldn't dilute Noni with some low cost fruit juice. But you can do that if you can't stand the taste.

Potassium – Potassium is a major mineral as well as an electrolyte; which means it carries an electrical charge. This positive charge ensures the Potassium is able to perform all of its necessary body functions. It also ensures that your muscles, including your heart, are able to contract and relax properly. Every fluid in your body contains Potassium, of which about 95% of that is found in your cells. Potassium and sodium work together to maintain things such as muscle tone, water balance and blood pressure. Too much sodium can deplete the body's Potassium. This balance is the job of your kidneys.

The presence of Potassium in your body helps to control the balance of fluid in your cells and in your blood. Potassium also works with another electrolyte, called bicarbonate, to maintain the pH of your blood and acid-base balance in your body. Potassium helps regulate the amounts of the minerals, calcium and phosphorus in your blood and prevents your bones and kidneys from excreting too much of these minerals. Because of this regulation, Potassium ensures that your bones stay dense and strong.

Potassium helps the body excrete a substance called citrate. If the body contains too much citrate, it can bind with calcium and form calcium citrate kidney stones. Because Potassium helps excrete citrate, it can lower your risk of developing kidney stones.

Controlling your Potassium is a major problem with kidney patients. High Potassium in the blood is called hyperkalemia. Low Potassium (hypokalemia) is rarely a problem for people with advanced kidney failure, because the kidney loses the ability to remove Potassium. To keep your Potassium down, avoid beans and peas; especially green beans. Eight ounces of green beans has the same amount of Potassium as 3 or 4 medium size oranges or bananas. For more information, refer back to **Kidney disease** in Chapter 8.

There is Potassium in every living food item you consume; meat, fruit, vegetable, nuts and berries. Even a lot of processed food products have Potassium additives. So Potassium supplements are not recommended, unless a doctor specifically instructs you to do so.

Sage – Sage is originally from the Mediterranean region but is widely grown in sunny locations with well-drained soil. Sage is known for its flavor on turkey and turkey stuffing. Sage has always been a "cure all" among Native Americans. Sage has also been used for sore throats, eye infections, gum disease, weak appetite, menopausal hot flashes and excessive sweating, infertility, tonsillitis, mouth sores and ulcers. Sage is used externally for wounds and ulcers.

In general, Sage is an astringent, antiseptic, antispasmodic, bitter tonic and stimulant. Sage is used as a throat and mouth wash you use by making a strong tea and gargling with it.

For ages, sage has been used in treatments for disorders involving the gastrointestinal tract. Sage helps to relieve muscle spasms in the digestive region and it is also been used as a cure for indigestion. It has also been known to help lower blood sugar levels in diabetics. It is also a fact that sage helps to improve memory and brain function. When used in combination with rosemary and ginkgo biloba, it is thought to help prevent and even slow down the progression of Alzheimer's.

Grow your own herbs and include Sage, so that you will have fresh live Sage to use to provide the health benefits it is known to provide you. Cut the Sage and dry it at the end the growing season. Cut the plant back to about one third its size and hang the branches upside down and bundled together. Once it dries naturally in a few days, strip the leaves off the branches and store it in vacuum sealed jars, bags or canisters. Make sure to add some Sage to your soups and stews too.

What did I leave out? I left out a lot of Vitamins and herbs because this is not a book about teaching you about what Vitamins and herbs are. I didn't go into all the little extra poisons in your food drinks and water, for this same reason. Almost all the information in this chapter are facts known for centuries to thousands of years. I only included this chapter as a convenience so that you could look in this book and find out about the major Vitamins, Herbs and Healing Foods I talk about which are needed to cure you.

My goal with this book is to give you information that is scarcely available and never talked about in the media. I have medical books and books on health and nutrition. And only a rare few have much of the information in this book.

I didn't want to get off on a long drawn out tangent. The focus needs to stay on recognizing all the major poisons and avoiding them and correcting your diet deficiencies to bring your cure to fruition. Do your research on everything you put in your body. Know what you are REALLY putting in your body.

Also, any food substance you can find that is live, whether it's wheat grass, sprouts or any plant food, as long as it's alive it has real value. All live food nourishes our bodies. So remember this when you are wondering IF you should buy a food product. Every lifeless food you eat instead of live plants with all those life-giving enzymes will not really help you with your cures.

And when you can, juice some fruits and/or vegetables. The fastest way to kill yourself is by regularly consuming liquid poisons like sodas and fruit juices. This is because in liquid form, your body absorbs them faster and in greater amounts. But lucky for you, when you juice produce, your body absorbs that juiced produce faster and in bigger amounts. And juicing is the next best thing to eating live produce and plant foods.

My recommendation is to stick with eating as much live fresh produce as you can and juice as often as it is convenient. If you try to have a diet of just juicing, you will lose the benefits of all the nutrients and fiber in that produce you juice. Doing both are of tremendous value for any cure and a long term solution for staying healthy and free of disease!

Now I will give you specific information to cure cancer.

10 - THE CURE FOR CANCER

One of the most feared diseases is cancer. But it is also one of the easiest to cure. So I want to take cancer and tell you all I can to help you get yourself cured. In the next chapter I do the same thing with the deadliest disease of all, chronic kidney disease. Besides giving you the cure to cancer and all disease in this book, I help you adjust your mind and attitude back to normal so that you can cure yourself. It's like I've already said, that nowhere in this country are doctors talking about curing anyone. And as a result, none of you ever talk about cures amongst yourselves!

It is this perverted state of mind that MUST be dealt with if you are to cure yourself and then remain cured. The saturation of poisons in our food, drinks and water supplies have to be dealt with or there is not much chance of you curing yourselves. Simply put, your current ways made you sick. And there is NO chance of that changing unless you change your way of thinking about what you eat and drink and stop believing the FDA's vulgar nonsense about poisons being safe! Poisons are the causer of 80% of all disease! Now can't you accept the fact that is NOT true?

So I talk about these attitudes, because it's these attitude adjustments that will change your way of thinking and change your life for the better. I know how scared you are. I know how terrified I was when suddenly I was given just 2 or 3 years to live. Listening to doctors will never get you cured. But I know that if you do what this book says, you are definitely going to cure yourself of cancer and ALL diseases, just as I did! And you will know that too about 2-3 weeks after you start doing what this book says to do; starting with drinking the baking soda water, taking Vitamin C, Fish and/or Flax seed oil and Magnesium.

The rest of this chapter is the information you need to cure yourself of cancer. So all those of you with cancer can get ready to end that cancer now. I don't care if the doctors gave you just weeks to live. You CAN be cured and will be cured if you do what this book says to do. Drinking the baking soda water will cause your cancer to be unable to survive in your body any longer. And with all this other great help, curing yourself is almost certain. I can't guarantee you that you will repair all the damage your cancer has done to your body. But curing your cancer will bring an end to the possibility of you dying from cancer.

Laying the Foundation for your cure. Yes, there is a cure for cancer. But like all cures, the cure for cancer is outside the helpless medical profession. The cure for cancer is not a gimmick. The cure for cancer is proven science that all doctors COULD tell you but don't. Your doctor only cares about prolonging your illness to maximize his income. But almost all of you will say that your doctor is different and that he or she really cares! OK, I'll play along. But let's get some proof that your doctor really cares.

If your doctor cares, he would have told you what caused your cancer. Here's how that caring doctor conversation went. Your doctor told you that your cancer was caused by poisons and told you this:

Cancer is caused by damage to the nucleus of cells. This damage interferes with apoptosis, which is the natural programmed death of cells. When this process breaks down, cancer cells begin to form. Cancer cells do not experience programmed death as normal cells do. This allows cancer cells to grow and divide, which leads to a mass of abnormal cells that grows out of control and forms tumors.

Once these tumors form, they develop blood vessels. These blood vessels carry cancer cells to other parts of the body and form growths. The damage to cells is caused by gene mutations causing cells to be unable to correct DNA damage. Cancer is a result of these mutations which interfere with oncogene and tumor suppression gene function and leads to this uncontrollable cell growth. Carcinogens are directly responsible for damaging DNA and promoting cancer. Free radicals are formed when our bodies are exposed to carcinogens. These free radicals damage cells and inhibit normal cell function.

If your family members, especially your parents and grandparents, have had cancer, it's obvious this gene mutation was passed on to you. But even so, this only means cancer forms quicker in these people than those without the family history of cancer. And as soon as your body is exposed to carcinogens, cancer begins to form. So, you can easily see how **avoiding poisons is the key to preventing and curing cancer. This is why all cancer patients should get serious about avoiding and eliminating poisons.**

Yep, that's what your doctor explained to you didn't he! No he didn't. Because he would lose a lot of money by telling you this. Poisons caused your cancer. And no doctor is going to tell you that, beyond mentioning cigarettes and alcohol, because doctors know that if you stop poisoning yourself, your cancer is going to fade away! So doctors have all these ways to "treat" your cancer and the symptoms that come with cancer. But no doctor is ever going to cure you of cancer or anything.

You might want to explain to yourself WHY you think doctors COULD cure you, when no doctor has ever studied cures in medical school. As a matter of fact, and I do mean fact, doctors don't even practice medicine nowadays. But is all this about doctors going to cure you? Answer – NO!

What this talk about doctors is for, is to adjust your attitude that made you sick in the first place. And if you don't get your attitude adjusted to the realities of science and facts, then you only need to make sure your funeral coverage is paid up to date. And even IF doctors told you the cure for cancer, as I am going to do, they still couldn't cure you. And neither can I! But I know someone who

CAN cure you. And it's the same person that made you sick in the first place.........YOU! Yes YOU are the one who can cure YOU.

YOU can learn to face the fact that poisons are NOT safe, no matter how often the FDA tells you they are certified "safe". Your parents told you poisons were bad for you. But you got all grown up and told everybody that you will do as you please and that nobody is going to tell you what you CAN and can NOT eat! But **you forgot to tell yourself that YOU are the one who is going to have the cancer and other chronic diseases those poisons cause.**

So now it's time for YOU to clean your mess up and get to thinking outside that tiny bubble where you trusted your government and the corporations, all the way to cancer or some other chronic disease or diseases! Diseases are only chronic because you trust doctors with no cures to cure you! Pretty crazy, huh? I mean really, do you take your car to the grocery store to have a new muffler put on? No you don't! So why are you going to doctors for cures, when doctors have no cures and didn't even study cures in medical school!

The cure for cancer is easy to understand and follow. But **you can't cure yourself as long as you are waiting on doctors and the medical profession to find the cures for cancer that already exist!** But plenty of you will walk for the cure for cancer, share cancer posts on Facebook in support of finding the cures for cancer that already exists. But the thing you never ever do is, share the cure for cancer with others!

In the city I live in, there's all the big buzz about the new cancer "care" center they are building. And boy do doctors CARE about cancer. Yep, doctors care about keeping your cancer around so they can maximize their income off your suffering and pain, instead of telling you how to cure yourself of cancer. But there will never ever be a cancer CURE center in this town! Everything has to be filtered through money. Cures help people and save their lives. But cures take millions and billions of dollars of income from the medical profession. That's why all cures are Dead On Arrival with doctors and the medical profession. And until cures start being taught in medical school, cures have no chance of being a part of the work of doctors and the medical profession.

So you have got to decide IF you want to live. And if you do, you can go ahead and cure yourself WHILE you still go to the doctor and follow all the quackery they have invented over the past 75 years, as doctors and the medical profession turned their backs on all cures and all medicine ever known to man.

Do you understand that 100% of the drugs your doctors prescribe you are removed naturally by your body? Your body begins to remove all drugs the moment they enter the body. That's why you have to keep taking them every day. But if doctors used real medicines, your body would put those real medicines to use in your body and only remove a small part of that real medicine. So am I saying to NOT take the drugs doctors prescribe you?

NO, I am not. What I am saying is that even the drugs your doctors prescribe you that do help you in some temporary way, are still poisons to your body that have to be completely removed. And to do that, your body uses up its own energy. Let me explain this a little more.

Your body only has so much energy. Your body needs energy to digest food, remove toxins, perform body metabolisms and repair damaged cells. You have got to learn to force your body to spend as much of its energy repairing damaged cells as you possibly can. Remember, cancer is caused by poisons damaging the nucleus of cells; which prevents the natural programmed death of cells. But if you stop stuffing those poisons down your throat, there won't be any poisons to cause cancer or any other chronic diseases!

I had a nice awakening to these scientific facts shortly after doctors told me I would be dead from chronic kidney disease by 2008 or 2009. I was talking to a nurse at the hospital and she mentioned that her husband had chronic kidney disease. I asked her what he was doing for his kidney disease. She said he was using ginger packs placed on his back next to his kidneys and that those ginger packs were soaking the poisons out of his kidneys.

Now when she told me this, I got all excited and couldn't wait to start using the ginger packs to get those poisons out of me. But as I was trying to track down the ginger roots, I started thinking...... now what if I don't put those poisons IN my body in the first place. Then there would be no need to soak them OUT of my kidneys! And that got my head to thinking a 100 miles an hour!

I started examining everything I ate and drank and everything my body comes in contact with; all the way from the food I eat, the water I drink and bathe in and the personal hygiene items we all use, like soap, shampoo, conditioner and my underarm deodorants. And even though I have been an Organic Gardener for the past 30 years, I still saturated my kidneys with so much poison in my drinks that they failed.

Lots of people said "Watch what you eat". But no one ever said "Watch what you DRINK" or "Watch what you shower in". And not doing that is what took out my kidneys after having arthritis, bleeding gums, intestinal bleeding and acid reflux for 20 years; not to mention all the headaches I had all my life. I cured myself of all that and more. And I did it all without any help from doctors.

As a matter of fact, I cured myself of every chronic disease and medical condition I had, by doing what I told you in the chapters called Poisons in Your Water, Poisons in Your Drinks and Poisons in Your Food. But when it comes to trying to stop exposing your body to poisons for a disease like cancer, you need to look beyond your food, drinks, water and hygiene items.

There are so many poisons and so many ways to become exposed to those poisons. That exposure can occur at your work place, play or other normal activities we all participate in. It can be the toxic foods all schools serve children, your garden supplies like pesticides, fungicides and fertilizers, working in a manufacturing plant or at food and drink corporations where they make these poisons that saturate the entire food and drinks supplies.

The constant principle that you MUST learn and understand, is that poisons cause ALL disease, except for the 20% caused by germs and viruses. And that by eliminating the poisons that caused the cancer in the first place, will cause the cancer to fade away naturally. This is the proven science that cures you. And this same proven science is the cure for every disease known to man. Without the poisons, there can be no disease. There can be NO cancer. But when most people hear these proven facts of science, they claim that they haven't been exposed to any real poisons. And that is where I have to point out the pride crushing facts about what a fool you really are. And I don't mean that in a mean way.

I rode the ship of fools until just a few years ago. So I don't have much room to talk. But I have abandoned the ship of fools through proven science which no doctor is willing to tell you. When I had bladder stones during the mid-90's, it is science that dictates that Magnesium dissolves calcium and that bladder stones (and kidney stones and bone spurs) are formed by particles of calcium combining with toxins to form bladder and kidney stones. So I took Magnesium oxide tablets and stopped my 4th bladder stone attack within an hour of it beginning and have not had a bladder stone attack since then, 1996; which is 17 years as of now.

I could have learned all this BEFORE my 4th bladder stone attack. But I didn't. And that ignorance caused me a lot of pain and money! Doctors said there was no cure for bladder stones either. And when I called them to tell them I would pay all the UN-necessary tests and hospital bills if they would tell me the cure for bladder stones, what I got was threats. They threatened to call the Police and have me arrested if I didn't stop asking them for the cure. They even called me the devil. I told them "OK, I'm the devil and you're calling the Police to have me arrested. But could you give me the cure for bladder stones?" But this only made them more irate!

This was after my 3rd bladder stone attack. And when the 4th one came, I was not going to consider the $1000+ ER bill and no cure I already got from them. And I sure the heck wasn't going to ask a damn doctor for a cure again and get called the devil and threatened with being arrested for it! So I took 2 250mg Magnesium oxide tablets 30 minutes into my 4th bladder stone attack. And within an hour, the attack subsided and faded away. And that was THE END of bladder stone attacks in my life. Science works and keeps on working!

When it comes to curing cancer, at first you might think that curing cancer is a whole lot harder than curing chronic kidney disease. And you would be wrong by a long shot. Everyone who gets chronic kidney disease, dies from it. A rare rare few get transplants that spare their lives. But since that transplanted kidney goes into that same person that already poisoned their kidneys into failure, they do the same thing to the new, healthy, transplanted kidney.

Without a lifestyle and diet change, no cure is possible. You have to choose whether you want to live OR you want to keep eating at restaurants, swigging sodas, eating red meat, cooking with the microwave, soaking your body with chlorine and filling your lungs with chlorine gas in the shower and a host of other bad habits that lead to sickness and a sure death, with no hope of getting better. It's very rare when it's just one poison that causes your chronic disease.

It's the overloading of poisons that creates sickness in your body. Let me give you a rundown of the huge amounts of poisons we all consume without any thought. Let's run through a day in most people's lives and stop to talk about it, every time your body is being poisoned. But before we do that, I need to cover just a few more things. You will see how this all fits together once you are finished reading this part of this chapter.

It's doing the things in the chapters about poisons in your food, drinks and water that ARE the cure for cancer and the cure for any disease that ails or afflicts you. These chapters contain the information you will use on a daily basis as you learn to recognize poisons in order to avoid them. What I am doing now, is telling you the other things you need to know in order to make cures a reality for you and in your life.

Cures are not a part of your life. You have always depended on doctors to fix the damage you do to your own body by ignoring science. That science has manifested itself as disease in your body. What I am teaching you is how to cause cures to manifest themselves in your body. And the first question you might have is "how is my body going to heal itself?" or "Can my body really heal itself of cancer?" The answer is YES! You already have the proof of that. But what am I talking about?

You have cut your finger before, right? You still have that cut? No! Well! I guess your body does heal itself. But even though all cuts you have ever had have healed and gone away, you didn't even know to put Vitamin E on those cuts to make them heal 3 times as fast and fade the scars much faster. But that science was always there, even when you had never heard of that. And the science to cure your cancer exists now, and has existed all along. But the cure for cancer and the cure for every disease has gained a vicious added element.

So what use to cure cancer will no longer cure cancer. And that element is the saturation of addicting, poisons (drugs, chemicals, toxins) that corporations put in all their products. And the leading poison is high fructose corn syrup.

There is no worse disease causing substance than high fructose corn syrup. It's in everything. And when I say everything, I MEAN.... everything. It's in your bread and everything sweet. And it's the main ingredient in countless Bar-BQ sauces, ketchups, salad dressings and things like that. You have one choice of each of those items that are not saturated with HFCS. The worst things you can put in your body are soda pops and fruit juices. I explained this in the chapter about Poisons in Your Drinks. I also explained how you are fooled by lying labels and catch phrases that never mean what they say and the gimmicks of labeling products "low fat", "low sodium", "reduced calories", "All Natural" and other complete nonsense corporations use to trick you into continuing buying their poison saturated products under the guise of being healthy.

Earlier, I told you we would take a look into a typical person's day and stop to talk about the poisons you come in contact with during normal daily activities. Let's do that right now.

OK, you just got a good night's sleep. The alarm clock goes off. You hit the snooze button and get up 10 minutes later when the snooze goes off. Time to hit the bathroom for a shit, shower and shave or a wee wee! Ahh, you get into the shower and it hits you - that warm water all over your body making you feel good and stimulating you to wake on up. But what else is going on?

You are soaking your entire body, filling and soaking every pore on your body with deadly chlorine. Yea, chlorine is deadly. Hitler used it to murder millions of people in WW II. Yea, it's no secret. But you have kept this scientific fact out of your mind and thinking. It's time to wake up. That chlorine kills the oxygen in every cell it comes into contact with and also kills the oils in your skin and scalp. Now why would you have dandruff (dry scalp) by soaking your entire head and body with oxygen killing chlorine!

And you stand there in the shower playing Nazi against yourself; breathing in that hot water vapor with all that chlorine gas mixed in it! Gee! I can't figure out why that happens unless ......unless ...yea, I hope you guessed it, unless you include proven science in your thinking. Then you won't soak your entire body in chlorine and fluoride WHILE gassing yourselves with chlorine gas. But wait, you just got up to start your day and that's just the shower.

So you get out of the shower and dry off with a chemically treated bath towel. Then soak your underarms with poisonous aluminum-zirconium or some other aluminum compound you can't pronounce. That harms your lymph nodes, which are your back up immune system. So, am I telling you to stop taking a shower and using underarm deodorants? NO. Read the chapter titled Poisons in Your Water and you'll know the solutions to these problems.

Then after saturating your body and lungs with deadly chlorine, you soak your underarms with toxic poisons and go to the table to have your breakfast. You sit down to eat some eggs, bacon, toast and coffee maybe. But what is that crap you are eating? All of it is acidic. That white bread toast is all poison. Your bacon and eggs have some nutritional value, but are soaked in chemicals from the feed the chicken and hogs eat; not to mention how hogs eat their own feces. Any acidic substance you put in your body inhibits normal body metabolisms. And the coffee is acidic too. That milk and sugar you put in your coffee are acidic. The milk has growth hormones, antibiotics and other drugs milk cows are routinely injected with. And the sugar is pure poison. Sugar is a drug, not a food substance. Same is true of white flour. They're all drugs. Sugar has the same effect on your brain as cocaine does. (More on this later) Now it's time to go to work.

Now, you know more about your work places than I do. So I want you to take the time to write this part of the book with all the work places you work in and all the obvious dangers and exposures to chemicals, dust and other toxins in your work places. And add those to all the stuff I have been telling you. But while you're at work, you most likely will eat that sugary crap and drink pure poison drinks at your work place at lunch and during breaks.

And add the poisons you consume when you eat out at a restaurant for lunch. There's no healthy food or drinks at restaurants. The game to addict you to their food is just as intense as what you get from corporations in the grocery store and on TV. Poisoning you is Right and Safe, because the government says so! And the corporations laugh all the way to the bank. And your doctors follow behind them in squeezing as much money out of you as they can, for the consequences of what the corporations caused in the first place. What a heinous racket! Then it's time to go home and eat supper.

Most people eat a pretty good supper. But most people have red meat and potatoes and tea. Pretty good eating, huh? Nope, not really. Once again you have the growth hormones, antibiotics and all the other drugs beef cattle are injected with and the poison soaked dead food they are fed. And, you are eating their dead flesh! Oh well, those potatoes are pretty good for you, as long as you peel the poison soaked skin off of them, or at least scrub them with a steel brush! Then you boil them to leech out most of the nutrients. Then pour that water down the drain. The tea helps fight cancer and the lemon slice too. Then the sugar in the tea is still pure poison.

Now it's time to go brush your teeth again and soak your mouth with a host of chemicals. And maybe through the day, I took an antacid, Aleve or Tylenol. And I have a prescription or two I have to take. And all of it is poisons that your body has to remove. That uses valuable energy. And now you're off to bed, to start this cycle over again.

Now add all those poisons up and you'll have no problem seeing WHY you have cancer or any other diseases! And I didn't even count any snacks, cigarettes, alcohol or recreational drugs lots of people consume.

Now an extremely important thing you should do is use an inexpensive, common substance. It's almost silly what this substance is. It reverses the acidic condition that allowed your cancer to survive and thrive in your body in the first place. **Cancer can NOT, I repeat, can NOT, live in an alkaline**

environment. This common item is none other than baking soda, sodium bicarbonate; also called meetha soda. Cancer cells are also more acidic than the cells around the cancer.

Baking soda is pH 14 and when mixed with water makes the entire glass of water become a pH of 8.0-8-5. It can be more if you use a carbon water filter and slightly higher if you use an osmosis system or fluoride filter. Merely mixing 1/2 teaspoon baking soda in 4-6 ounces of water and drinking at least twice daily, before bed and when you awake, will serve as the foundation for your near certain cure. You should drink it 3-5x daily.

Baking soda reverses the acidic state of your body that made it possible for you to develop chronic disease and for disease to survive in your body. So make sure you keep plenty of baking soda around. And make sure to drink 1/2 teaspoon baking soda with 4-6 ounces of water at least 2x daily, as the start and foundation of curing every disease you have and preventing disease from developing in the first place.

The only precautions I know to tell you about baking soda is that prolonged excess use can make your body too alkaline. Also, use baking soda only at the minimum suggested dose and length of time if you have a problem with excess salt. Baking soda is sodium bicarbonate. So it can raise your blood salt levels.

It actually lowered my salt. That was the first scientific proof of a theory I had about your body seeing excess acid as salt. Your kidneys retain extra water to dilute acid just like salt. As the baking soda neutralizes acid, your kidneys remove that excess water it had retained to dilute that acid, same as salt. I am excited about what this means and the results I am now getting.

You would be well served to find a book by Dr. Mark Sircus tilted simply "Sodium Bicarbonate – Full Medical Review", 2nd edition; a book I only recently found out about. Dr. Sircus also has 2 books about curing cancer.

The near miraculous effects of sodium bicarbonate are explained in Dr. Sircus' book. Baking soda will relieve heartburn instantly. It also cures metabolic acidosis of your kidneys which causes almost all chronic kidney disease and gets you well on your way to curing yourself of CKD.

You can even brush your teeth with it. Just wet your toothbrush. Shake it off once or twice. Then dip it in a box of baking soda to cover your brush with baking soda. Then brush and slosh the liquid around in your mouth a bit. This will neutralize the acid on your teeth and gums and stop most tooth pain and lessen the severity of sensitivity to heat and cold. Wherever you need to kill fungus or neutralize an acidic substance, call baking soda to the rescue!

There are so many things baking soda is good for. Some of its uses are that it absorbs radiation, alkalizes the body, absorbs heavy metals, treats colds and the flu, treats insect bites and itchy skin, soothes your feet and is a non-toxic deodorant. You can also use it to clean many things like dishes, floors, furniture, shower curtains, baby clothes and cloth diapers, cars, batteries, combs and brushes and to clean the dirt and residue off fresh produce; as well as clean your bath tub, tile and sinks. Baking soda can also be used as a facial scrub and body exfoliant, to freshen linens, deodorize stinky feet or make a bath soak.

Although all of those uses are great, the lifesaving value of baking soda is the most important. It absorbs radiation, in case of a nuclear attack or exposure such as chemotherapy and radiation.

And don't be fooled by the medical profession. They use sodium bicarbonate to keep chemotherapy and radiation patients from dying from the toxicity of their chemical drugs and for clinical acidosis in patients. It's a vile story about why they stick with their dangerous expensive chemicals in spite of knowing safe, inexpensive natural medicinal solutions. It's all about greed and it is greed with no thought of what is good for you, the patient!

As we go to the next part to learn the things you have to know to improve your health on the way to your cures, remember that unless you believe you CAN be cured, it's never going to happen. I do NOT mean mind over matter or something stupid. I mean that cures are not a part of your thinking, much less your life. In this country we have faith in our doctors that there ARE no cures for any diseases. We have crawled into that helpless bubble over the past 75 years.

But because of people like me that know there are cures for every disease and have cured ourselves of what doctors call "incurable" diseases, we're gonna tell you the Truth about the cures and do everything we can to get this information to you. The hope is that cures will return to being a part of lives, communities and countries for the Protection, Welfare and Benefit of The People. But do NOT pretend that the helpless state of this country's sick care, health care system, is of The People, by The People or For The People.

Let's Get You Started on Getting Rid of Your Cancer

This is where you start learning the things that will directly affect your cancer and train your body to heal itself. Still, there are no gimmicks. We are learning how to use science to heal our bodies and how to speed that healing as much as we possibly can. You will need to use chapters 5, 6 & 7 as your daily guide in getting rid of the saturation of poisons in your food, drinks and water supplies.

But what I have told you so far is about attitude, state of mind; awakening to the fact that there IS a cure and you CAN be cured. You are going to cure yourself. And if you fall short, the least you will do is significantly improve your health and learn how to maintain that great improvement in your health.

I am not claiming to be some omnipotent, know it all. So there are so many different sets of circumstances in all the different people's lives. The one thing that does NOT change is science and its Laws of Physics. And that's why, if you do what this book says, you will certainly get the results stated. And for the skeptics and naysayers, I can only quote My Cousin Vinny if you wanna claim these Laws of Science do NOT work for you. And that's "Are we supposed to believe that the Laws of Physics cease to exist at your house!" So do the things in this book WHILE you still go along with your doctors; except for the parts about Death and dying and there's no cure.

One of the major things you have to do, is start drinking lots of pure filtered water. That's why the chapter called Poisons in Your Water came before the information about your food and drinks. Your body is 80% water. And it ain't 80% water-chlorine and fluoride. So your body has to work to remove 100% of the chlorine and fluoride in your water. Drink 1-ounce of water for every 2 pounds of body weight. And try to use pH drops to raise the alkalinity of your drinking water. You can get pH drops on Ebay. One side effect of the highly alkaline water will be weight loss. As the highly alkaline water neutralizes acid in your body, your kidneys will remove all that water it retained to dilute that acid, as a natural defense to that acid. That is how you lose the weight.

Your water needs to be filtered. A carbon water filter only filters out about 90% of the chlorine and nothing else. So that's why you need a fluoride water filter at least. A reverse osmosis filter system is better and filters all your water in your home. Using either of these water filters takes all the taste out of your water that you taste in tap water. The chemicals are bitter and acidic. So by removing chlorine and fluoride, the bitter acidic taste is gone and your water is alkaline. To increase the alkalinity of your water, add pH drops to your drinking water every day. This raises the pH to around 7.5-8.0 and above.

Flushing your kidneys with this highly alkaline water will neutralize acid and slowly transform your body's acidic state back into the normal alkaline state your body is supposed to be in. Your body became acidic over time as you consumed more and more animal products, sugar and chlorinated water. And the highly alkaline water reverses that disease ripe acidic environment inside your body. Chlorine destroys the oxygen in every cell it comes into contact with and kills the beneficial bacteria in your stomach and intestines. And your intestines are the central part of your immune system! Without your body being in this acidic state from consuming chlorinated water, sugars and animal products, your cancer would never have become a chronic disease.

You have to remember that your body is always making cancer cells. But when you overload your body and immune system with too many poisons for an extended period of time, your body is unable to remove cancer cells and other toxins as fast as they form. So they begin to gather in places in the body.

As cancer cells gather in your body, they will begin to cling to tissue and organs and begin to form blood vessels. This allows cancer cells to be carried to almost any place in your body. You've heard the doctors tell you this by saying "The cancer is spreading." So what can you do to arrest your cancer and send it into permanent remission, aka "cure"?

Start taking Vitamin C, Fish or Flax seed oil and Magnesium. Why? Because your diet is deficient in all of these. Why are Vitamin C, Fish or Flax seed oil and Magnesium so important?

First of all, this savage red meat "American diet" is insane to begin with. Men don't have the teeth for chewing meat. You need sharp fangs to cut and chew meat. We humans don't have sharp fangs. We are supposed to be on a fish diet, not this savage red meat diet. The Fish oil has the Omega-3 that your body must have or you develop diseases like arthritis, Alzheimer's, Parkinson's, heart disease, strokes and cancer. Flax seed oil is a vegetable source of Omega-3.

You need about 1000mg of Fish or Flax seed oil daily to maintain your health and prevent disease. You need 3-4 times that amount while you are sick. And try to eat fish as often as possible. Eat fish types that have scales like Cod, Tilapia, Salmon and Tuna. Catfish does NOT have scales.

Next, you need lots of Vitamin C. Why? Because Vitamin C is a common and readily available anti-oxidant. Anti-oxidants are the substances that remove toxins from your body. Your body does not store Vitamin C. So it is up to you to make sure you give your body a steady supply of Vitamin C. You should take at least 5000mg of Vitamin C daily if you have cancer. Taking more is better. Up to 10,000mg daily is what you should try to take. But increase your dose of daily Vitamin C gradually until you are at that level dosage.

You should also consider taking other anti-oxidants like Selenium, Beta-Carotene (Vitamin A), Vitamin E and other lesser known anti-oxidants. Vitamin E is a great way to speed repair to damaged cells both inside and out. You can find more information about most of these food substances in chapter 9.

But why do you have to take the magnesium? For one, Magnesium is needed to perform over 300 body metabolisms. Without sufficient Magnesium, these body functions don't occur. Add to that, the certain acidic state of your body which has already habitually inhibited all body metabolisms and you have a state of death settling into your body. And can you tell me where you are getting enough Magnesium in your diet? No you can't.

So take the Magnesium supplements; at least 250-400mg twice daily if you are sick or 250-400mg most days to maintain your health and prevent disease. I already told you that unless you take Magnesium vitamins, you are bound to form bladder or kidney stones and/or bone spurs. Correcting these major nutrient deficiencies in your diet will go a long way in your efforts to improve your health as you work toward your goal of being cured.

Once you do what I've told you so far, you will be on your way to reversing that acidic, disease ripe state of your body, begin to lose weight, begin to feel better almost every day and notice that your body is recovering within 3-4 weeks. That improvement will depend on how well you conform your food, drinks and water to what is told in chapters 5, 6 & 7 and how well you correct these major diet deficiencies. Let's take a look at a commonly known beverage that leads the way to many diseases and is bad for you in every way.

Now, a soda pop is a good example of how bad all those poisons are. People fool themselves by thinking that soda pop gives them a welcome energy boost! But it's no energy boost! What really happens is this: You begin drinking that high fructose corn syrup soaked soda in liquid form with that DNA altering sodium benzoate and that 3.0 acidic carbonated water. And your body goes into instant shock as it tries to defend itself against all that poison.

This instant elevated activity our bodies go into to remove these poisons is what we falsely tell ourselves is a harmless, healthy energy boost. And it takes your body up to 6 hours to remove the poisons in a 12-ounce soda pop. That cripples your immune system. And by drinking a 12-ounce soda every 6 hours, you in effect, nullify your immune system. And this is just one example of what you will learn in chapters 5, 6 & 7.

Fasting - Another major thing you can do to speed your healing is to fast. It is not necessary to fast for days. By simply eating your last meal around 6 PM, then not eating again until between 6 and 10 AM the next day, will do a lot for you; especially if you make it a habit. Fasting was the foundation of the medical practice of Hippocrates, the Father of Medicine.

What fasting does is to relieve the body of the most energy consuming bodily task of digesting food. Once your body ceases to digest food, your body then uses that energy to repair damaged cells in our bodies. And when you are sick, your body needs to use as much energy as possible to repair damaged cells and remove toxins. The less poisons you put into your body, the more energy your body has to use to remove those toxins.

Your body only has so much energy. It uses most of its energy to digest food. It uses the rest of its energy to remove toxins and repair damaged cells. So you have to learn how to make your body use more and more of its energy to repair damaged cells to heal and cure you. The easiest way to do that is to fast as often as possible and cut down on the amount of food you eat. Using chapters 5, 6 & 7 to reduce the amount of poisons you consume in your food, drinks and water, will relieve your body of having to use so much energy to remove toxins from your body.

Doing this and fasting allows your body to use most of its energy to repair damaged cells, which eventually results in you being cured.

No matter how long you can manage to fast, remember to drink plenty of pure water. If you go more than 2 or 3 days without food, don't hesitate to eat a bite of fruit or raw vegetables. Stuff like that aids in your healing and doesn't take much energy to digest.

But why hasn't your doctor told you to do this? Your doctors are the ones who swore an Oath to Hippocrates when they became "doctors". But they're not telling you about the main part and foundation of the Medical Practices of

Hippocrates, the Father of Medicine.

I have never sworn an Oath to Hippocrates. But I'm the one telling you "Do what the Father of Medicine did".

With 133,000,000 Americans who have at least one chronic disease, is that what you call the result of the best health care system in the world? Yes you do! But it's complete nonsense. Each of those 133,000,000 Americans represents a failure of this country's medical profession. Even with 10,000,000 Americans with chronic disease, we should have declared a national emergency.

But with 133,000,000 Americans with at least one chronic disease, we not only haven't declared a national emergency, we continue to declare that we have the best health care system on the planet! If every single person had at least one chronic disease, they would still tell you that! And you would still believe them! I don't know of any greater incompetence in any profession or line of work than this country's medical profession and health care system.

When I got those statistics above from the Center for Disease Control web site, http://www.cdc.gov/chronicdisease/overview/index.htm, I noticed their web site also talked about what causes these chronic diseases. But guess what they did NOT mention in that information? Not one word about poisons in your food, drinks and water supplies. The closest they came was naming cigarettes or alcohol as a cause of lung cancer or liver disease. Whoop dee Do!

But it's the same thing at the doctor's office! Rarely does a doctor tell you what caused your chronic disease. I have asked almost everyone I have talked to if their doctor has ever told them what caused their chronic disease. I never get any specific answers; just vague generalizations!

Now that's what you should be getting from rank amateurs, but NOT from professionals! A professional is assumed to be an expert in their field or occupation. But how can you call the medical profession that has failed to cure the diseases of over 133,000,000 people at this very moment, "experts"! Face reality as it is. With over 133,000,000 known cases of complete failure by this country's doctors and medical profession, it's well past time to try something new. You know, something that does NOT have over 133,000,000 known failures at any given moment!

People prefer to eat as much poisons as they choose and never think about what they're doing. They think they can run to the doctor and the doctor will save them from the consequences of their own actions. But what they end up with is one lifelong disease after another and a pile of prescriptions to take every day. You trust your food supply to be safe. You trust your drinks to be safe. You trust your water supplies to be safe. I've got some advice for you.

Stop trusting your food, drinks and water suppliers. What fluoride has to do with safe drinking water is a confusing scam that continues as I write.

Don't trust your water company and prove it by getting a water filter to protect yourself. You can afford a water filter. But you can't afford the medical bills that the chlorine and fluoride will burden you with. Again, it costs about $30-40 a year to prevent brittle bones, bladder cancer and a ravaged immune system; compared to the thousands to tens of thousands of $$$$$ in medical bills for treating the diseases caused by the chlorine and fluoride. You can afford the preventions, but not the treatments.

Again, stop trusting your food, drinks and water suppliers. I am not talking about the grocery stores either! The grocery store puts the garbage on the shelves that you buy again and again. If you didn't buy those poison soaked products, they would stop buying those products from their suppliers.

Grocery stores stock their shelves with products that sell the fastest. If only you were lucky enough to only be able to afford dry beans and brown rice!!!! And guess what? For the most part, the healthiest products are the cheapest. There are rare few exceptions. The most significant is with bread.

White bread is cheap, but has little to no real nutritional value; whereas whole wheat bread costs 3 times as much, but is highly nutritious. But since bread is a diet staple, you count on eating bread regularly. So it needs to be healthy and nutritious. Otherwise, you get the diseases and conditions white flour and white bread cause, starting with chronic diarrhea and intestinal bleeding. You can afford the cure, prevention. But you can't afford the treatments. The choice is yours to make. Just remember that it is you that has to make the changes.

One other major help in speeding you toward your cure is drinking Sage and/or Lemon Balm tea. Sage was a cure all to Indians. Still is. And Lemon Balm was a cure all to the Egyptians. I had a great experience drinking Lemon Balm tea when my kidneys failed. It sent healing warmth into every part of my insides it came into contact with. It was the only bright spot in the days of my worst nightmare. I know it works, same as Sage. One thing is that they have good amounts of anti-oxidants. You can find more information on Sage and Lemon Balm in chapter 9 - Vitamins, Herbs & Healing Foods.

You also have to understand that you need to eat as healthy a diet and drinks as you can. I mean, why drink a soda pop or fruit juice when you could drink something that your body doesn't have to work so hard to remove. You could drink fruit smoothies made with raw fruits. That would be almost 100% good for your body. Those live fruits and vegetables have enzymes that pump life into your body. And your body doesn't work to remove that live produce. Your body uses most of that live produce. And if you juice that produce, it's easier for your body to digest than solid food.

So it takes far less energy to digest that produce if you run them through a good juice making machine. But even if you don't juice or don't do it often, you can still try to eat as much raw fruits and vegetables as you possibly can.

As a matter of fact, **if you just get those water filters and follow what I call**

The Perfect Diet, you can cure yourself or significantly improve your health without having to learn how to read food labels and avoid the masses of products that are saturated with poisons; most of which we pretend are food. I laid out the simple Perfect Diet at the first of this book. The Perfect Diet is the best diet to be on. But since it is a far cry from the "American diet", you may do best by using chapters 6 & 7 to clean up your current diet that caused your diseases in the first place.

Chapters 6 & 7 are for cleaning up your present diet by beginning to avoid the saturation of poisons in our food and drinks supplies. This is what most of you need, because in my opinion, it's not practical to tell you that you have to become a vegetarian if you want to be cured. And that effort always starts with you accepting the facts that white flour, white sugar and high fructose corn syrup are drugs, NOT food! So the cure for cancer includes you doing what chapters 5, 6 & 7 guide you to do in cleaning up your current diet.

Some other things that help speed your healing along are what I am going to tell you about now. Read this book, then use chapters 6 & 7 to clean up the food and drinks you consume. Chapter 5 boils down to the details of why you need a water filter and a shower filter. All of this is an essential part of every cure and every prevention of chronic disease.

What else You Can Do To Speed Your Healing

I know that's a lot to take in about all the poisons in your water, drinks and food products and the obsession corporations have with deceiving you and addicting you to the chemicals they saturate all their products with. That is why I often told you to use chapters 5, 6 & 7 as a guide from now on. Judge your water, drinks and food according to what is stated in those chapters.

This book is about YOU being cured. YOU getting better. I'm not against doctors. I am FOR people and animals being well and staying free of disease.

I don't allow my thoughts to be filtered through money, religion, politics, opinions or anything else. I had to become that way to save my own life. Everything I shared in this book is to help you and help you return to making cures a part of Life, instead of remaining in that hopeless abyss under the helm of doctors with no cures and no natural medicine.

When it comes to doctors and this country's medical profession, they are the best doctors in the world in emergencies. But when it comes to disease, they are among the worst doctors in the world. And when you are dying, you don't have time to be distracted with a bunch of cold hearted greedy doctors. You have to focus on doing everything you can to get better and save your own life.

And even if this cure for cancer was not true, most of us believe that we don't just lay down and die. We try to live as long as we can and will fight as hard as we need to, in order to extend the time of our precious lives.

When I started doing these things myself, I didn't have a single thought of me curing myself of arthritis. Or a single thought about curing myself of heart disease. Or curing myself of headaches, heartburn, bleeding gums, intestinal bleeding or even dandruff! All I was trying to do was extend my life a little beyond the 2-3 years doctors gave me before I would be dead or on dialysis.

So I know you gotta be a bit skeptical that our food, drinks and water supplies are making us all sick and killing us years before our time. But it's true. And no corporation is going to remove those addicting poisons they saturate our food, drinks and water with.

It is all up to YOU to learn how to avoid their poisons. YOUR life depends on it. So you DO have the time to learn these things and save your own life. Then spread this knowledge to others until it spreads like wildfire, on the way back to normal thinking and way of living.

There are other things that are known to help people with cancer. But before I get to that, here's some specific information on cancer and breast cancer from other places in this book:

- **Breast Cancer** - Read the additional information about the cure for breast cancer on page 68 under this same heading **Breast Cancer.**
- **Cancer** – Read the additional information about the cure for Cancer on page 68, 69 and 70 under **Cancer** right after **Breast Cancer.**

Some other things that can help cancer patients are Astragalus, Vitamin C, Calcium, Calcium D-Glucarate, Cayenne, Vitamin D, Fish Oil, Flax seed Oil, Garlic, Lemon Balm and Sage.

Here's where you can take a closer look at these Vitamins, Herbs and Healing Food substances:

- **Astragalus** – Read about Astragalus on page 87 & 88 in chapter 9.
- **Vitamin C** – Read about Vitamin C on page 89 and view the Vitamin C dosage table on page 90.
- **Calcium** – Read about Calcium in chapter 9 on page 90 after the Vitamin C table.
- **Calcium D-Glucarate** – Read about Calcium D-Glucarate on page 90.
- **Cayenne** – Read about Cayenne on page 91.
- **Vitamin D** – Read about Vitamin D on page 91 also.
- **Fish oil** – Read about Fish oil on page 92 & 93 in chapter 9.
- **Flax seed** – Read about Flax seed oil on page 93 after **Fish oil.**
- **Garlic** – Read about Garlic on page 93 after **Flax seed.**
- **Lemon Balm** – Read about Lemon Balm on page 95.
- **Sage** – Read about Sage on page 99 & 100.

All of these Vitamins, Herbs and Healing Foods will add to your cure. So refer to the information for all these in chapter 9.

You should take as many additional anti-oxidants as you are willing to take. I don't mean huge doses. I mean, willing to take daily for a few months. Then continue taking them several times weekly the rest of your life. Some of the anti-oxidants besides Vitamin C are Vitamin E, Vitamin A, Selenium and Alpha Lipoic Acid. All of these remove the toxins that cause cancer. And Selenium is a very potent anti-cancer agent.

There are also large amounts of other anti-oxidants in Goji berries, Noni and Mangosteen. It is these extremely powerful anti-oxidants in high amounts that bring the claims of miracle healings by drinking the juices of Goji berries, as well as Mangosteen and Noni fruit. I highly recommend the pure forms of these. But you should never believe any ONE thing is going to cure you. It's the total amount of poisons that enter your body, not any ONE poison, or any ONE diet deficiency. Now, here's a short summary of what you should focus on eating.

The Best Things to Eat to Help Cure Cancer

Now that you have read what you have to know in order to cure yourself or at least significantly improve your health, I'll give you a short summary of what foods you should eat. This book focuses on reading labels to recognize the saturation of poisons in our food, drinks and water supplies, NOT a special diet you can follow to cure yourself. Technically, there isn't a special diet you can go on to cure any disease. Your diseases are caused by poisons. Anything that your body naturally removes is considered to be a toxin. That includes all man-made chemicals that enter your body through your mouth, nose, eyes, lungs, veins, pores or otherwise.

But there ARE foods that are more beneficial than others for people with cancer. Earlier in this book I told you what I consider to be The Perfect Diet. The Perfect Diet is the best diet for your overall best health. But to make sure you are eating the most beneficial foods for speeding your healing for cancer, here's what you should focus on:

Eat oily fish like salmon, herring and mackerel and others. Cat fish is not one of them. Cod and Tilapia are other good choices.

Stick to colorful fruits and vegetables such as carrots, peppers, pumpkins, cabbage, broccoli, Brussels sprouts, eggplant, tomatoes, apricots, cherries and red grapes. If the fruit or vegetable is purple, you can count on it being a strong agent against cancer.

Eat Mushrooms, Garlic, lentils, chick peas, soya, Brazil nuts, Pumpkin seeds and Sunflower seeds. All of these inhibit cancer cell growth, protects the immune system from toxins and stops the spread of cancer.

As important as this information is, I chose to simplify it as much as I can. The big job is trying to find something to eat in the grocery store that is NOT packed with disease causing poisons. And when you do that, the grocery store becomes a very tiny tiny place. You are tempted to continue buying the same crap that made you sick and is taking your life away from you. It takes some hard work and time to make the transition from debauchery to caring about your own health and life.

Debauchery is defined as extreme indulgence in sensual pleasures. And that is exactly why you are sick. Food corporations work to addict you to their products by adding substances like high fructose corn syrup in excessive amounts to addict your brain to their products. It's an addiction that affects the brain the exact same way cocaine does. You sit in the kitchen smacking on that sugary snack, cake, cookies and pies; washing it down with soda pops or fruit juices. You're 30-100 pounds or more overweight. You know you shouldn't be eating that crap! So WHY ARE YOU?

That's how you behave when you are addicted. It's the behavior of people who are addicted to the saturation of poisons in whole milk too; addicted to the growth hormones, antibiotics and all the other drugs cows are routinely injected with. Not to mention the poisons in that dead grain most cows are fed. You have got to face the fact that you are addicted to these poisons, so you can do something about it.

None of the food and drink corporations are going to remove their poisons. You have to deal with reality as it is; not how it SHOULD be. **If you're gonna depend on the corporations to remove the poisons that made you sick, then you have no hope whatsoever.** This book is about empowering YOU with the knowledge to cure yourself of cancer and all disease, by doing something to avoid the poisons that cause all disease. I don't want you to forget that your attitude and state of mind have to change before your health can change. I cannot cure you. And no doctor can cure you either.

YOU are the one who can cure YOU. And this book was written to provide you the information you must know in order to cure yourself, or at least significantly improve your health. You cannot eat those poisonous foods I just mentioned and expect to cure your cancer. It wasn't lack of fresh fruits and vegetables that made you sick. It was poisons, toxins, chemicals that made you sick. And the only way you are going to cure or prevent disease is by avoiding the poisons that cause all disease.

So this is the end of the information you need to cure yourself. But make sure you go ahead and read My Final Words about cancer next. I saved some interesting facts for the end of this chapter. And of course, there are other things that help cancer patients. But I have covered the knowledge and proven science that will cure you or at least improve your health significantly. I have said this more than once in this book. Why didn't I say everyone will be completely cured?

I don't know all the 100's of millions of circumstances in people's lives. So there is no way I can determine the outcome in ALL those people's lives. **What I**

can do and did do in this book is give you the written knowledge of proven science that man used throughout history to cure and prevent diseases. This is the information doctors began to intentionally ignore over the past 75 years, in order to prolong your illness to maximize their income.

But I did not waste my time trying to change doctors or the helpless medical profession! It's for that same reason I've said before - that poisons caused your disease, not lack of fruits and vegetables. And it wasn't for lack of doctors or nurses. And it wasn't caused by lack of exercise. Your cancer and all disease is caused by POISONS. **And since it's those poisons that cause all disease, it's those poisons you gotta concentrate on avoiding, in order for your health to recover and make you well again.**

Now that I have given you all the information you need to guide you in healing yourself as fast as you want to, I have a few things to tell you that I believe you need to be aware of. These are things about your cancer, all diseases, doctors and the medical profession, food and drink corporations and a few things about me and how I discovered the scientific cure for cancer. It's the information up to this point in the book that will save your life.

Before I end this part of the book about the cure for cancer, let me tell you a few more things that will help you with your cure. A more correct title would be A Cure For Cancer, since there are a few ways to cure yourself of cancer. This book tells you about the natural cure for cancer.

I will tell you about more cures for cancer here in:

My Final Words About Cures for cancer

Here we are at the end of the cure for cancer. I know you have learned a lot of things you did not know. The trick is to put the information to use so that your cure can be a reality and not just hope. I just can't stress it enough about poisons causing your diseases! So buying all the cancer diet books can help, but they are not the cure for cancer. The cure for cancer is to get rid of the CAUSE of all cancer. And the cause of all cancer is poisons.

It's like your floor being flooded with water. If you're a doctor, you charge us to mop up the water again and again. But a plumber finds the CAUSE of the leak and fixes the CAUSE of the leak in order to stop the consequences of the leak. So I cannot take credit for this common sense fact that we all know as humans. Find the cause. **Get rid of the cause and you get rid of the problem, the disease.** But how is it that I know the cure for cancer?

After doctors told me I would be dead or on dialysis by 2008 and would not do anything to help me get better, much less cure me, I started looking for anything that MIGHT help my kidneys get better. I had arthritis, bleeding gums, intestinal bleeding, headaches, heartburn and a few other diseases for at least 20 years. I had headaches from time to time my whole life. So I sure never gave one second of thought to curing myself of any of those conditions.

All I was trying to do was help my kidneys and hope I could add some time on to the short time I had left to live. And even after curing myself of chronic bladder stones in 1996, what I was about to do would end up shocking even me! It all began when my 84 year old mother was in Intensive Care in St Bernard's hospital.

I was talking to the head nurse in the Intensive Care wing at St. Bernard's, when she told me her husband also had kidney disease. I asked her what he was doing about it. She told me he was using ginger packs placed on his kidney area. These ginger packs soak poisons out of the kidneys. And since no one had told me anything that could help me, I was anxious to get some ginger root and start using these ginger packs.

But as I was looking for the ginger roots, I began thinking that you wouldn't have to soak the poisons OUT of your kidneys, if you didn't put those poisons IN your kidneys in the first place. Then, I wondered why anyone would put poisons IN their bodies in the first place. I also wondered what and where the poisons were coming from that caused my chronic kidney disease. And the intense search and activities began!

I began to examine everything I ate, drank or came into contact with. The first thing I did was buy a fluoride water filter to replace our Water Pik faucet end filter. Then I bought a shower filter. I also quit using the microwave to cook and began using it only to heat things up for 30 seconds or less. I couldn't find much wrong with what I was eating, except for some red meat. But when I began to examine what I was DRINKING, boy did the scum rise to the top in plain view!

And once I found that damned high fructose corn syrup saturating my fruit juices and soda pops, I began finding it in almost everything. I did some tests to see what was causing me to get all tense. And I kept getting that tense feeling every time I consumed something with high fructose corn syrup in it. And the more high fructose corn syrup a product had, the more tense it made me.

So I began avoiding the products with high fructose corn syrup in them. There goes my Kraft Bar-BQ sauces, mayonnaise, ketchup, ice cream, bread and on and on and on. Boy, when you begin to look, you soon learn that once you get rid of the products saturated with high fructose corn syrup, there's barely anything left in the grocery store you CAN buy.

And now, the heartless bastards that make this poison are running commercials claiming your body sees high fructose the same as sugar. My response is "My body never did. Your high fructose corn syrup almost killed me." And I am not looking for revenge against these killers. I am looking to save people from these killers and their saturation of addicting drugs they saturate all their products with.

Their response is to claim their products are safe like the FDA says. And that normal use of their products will not make you sick or kill you. But then you have THEM as the proof that they work hard and spend billions of dollars in advertising to entice you to consume large amounts of their poison saturated products! And the rare times "government" does their job to govern these poison peddlers, you have all these whackos claiming their Rights are being violated by the government not allowing them to buy excessive amounts of these corporations' poisons!

Now ordinarily, I would agree when government prevents you from doing something you choose. But when the City of New York banned sugary drinks over 16 ounces, they were not violating anyone's Rights. They were and are, forcing these poison peddling corporations to stop pushing their poison saturated drinks on the people in excessive amounts. The wrongs of these corporations are being limited, or governed, for the safety and well-being of The People. And this IS the real role of government.

The most important part of this is that, gene mutated high fructose corn syrup should already be banned. If it's just like any other sugar, then why is high fructose corn syrup the only sugar made from genetically altered corn and genetically altered enzymes?!?

Once I began to eliminate the high fructose corn syrup, things started changing for the better with me. It was the first thing I knew that was actually helping. And in this book, I have told you all the things I did to help myself and cure myself of chronic kidney disease and at least 7 other chronic diseases and medical conditions. That was every disease and medical condition I had. When all I was trying to do was help my kidneys get better to add a little time to my life, past the 2008-2009 time doctors said I would be dead or on dialysis.

I was so amazed at what happened, it took a while to sink in. I figured since there were no cures for any of these chronic incurable diseases I had, that I was probably just fooling myself while my diseases were actually getting worse.

But after a few years I began to accept the fact that I was actually cured of all those things. No more headaches, heartburn, arthritis, kidney problems, intestinal bleeding, bleeding gums or anything else. So as the days, weeks, months and a few years passed, it slowly began to sink in that I am actually cured of all this.

It's weird never having a headache. I haven't had a headache since early 2007, after having 2 or 3 a week for the past 20+ years; same as with the heartburn, bleeding gums, intestinal bleeding and arthritis.

I decided to write a book to share as much knowledge as I could, in order to help as many people as possible. The book focused on chronic kidney disease, but is titled "Self-Care Health Care Guide". I worked hard on that book and tried to keep it as a guide for curing yourself of everything I cured myself of.

Once I finished that book, I realized that book contained the cures for most diseases specifically. But even though the book was finished, I continued doing some research about other major diseases like cancer and liver disease and a few others. What I found out is that, one after another after another disease is caused by poisons.

Fact is, 80% of all disease is caused by poisons. The other 20% is caused by germs or viruses. All cancers are caused by poisons. But diseases such as hepatitis are caused by a virus. So I took those facts and back tracked them.

My books are about avoiding the poisons that cause all these chronic diseases. All cancers are caused by poisons. So there is your cure for cancer. I was really in shock for a few weeks and thought about all this over and over and over. And the more I thought about it, the more it excited me.

I wasn't looking for the cure for cancer, much less the cure for all chronic disease. But I lived it, THEN realized what I had actually done. It took me over a year to start thinking about writing this book, since I had already given the cures for every chronic disease in my first book, Self-Care Health Care Guide.

Never depend on the doctors or medical profession to cure you. Doctors never studied cures and never studied medicine either. As a matter of fact, doctors abandoned all cures and medicine in the entire history of man, starting about 75 years ago. Use doctors and the medical profession for what they DO. They're real good at doing tests and diagnosing disease, prescription drugs, surgeries, medical procedures and for emergencies. But when it comes to curing disease, the doctors in this country are among the worst in the world. This is why this nation's sick care "health care" system is only the 34th best care in the world, while being #1 in cost of that care.

So whether you listen to doctors or not, one thing is certain. The only way you have a chance of being cured is IF you cure yourself. Or maybe you think I have a chip on my shoulder just because this cure for cancer and most all disease is being ignored by the medical profession? My response to that would be "I'm not a 17 year old girl or a researcher at the University of Canada at Alberta either." So you might think "Terry, are you crazy? What does a 17 year old girl and researchers in Canada have to do with cures for cancer being ignored?"

Uh, I'm the one telling you the cure for cancer. But no one listens.

But no one is listening to 17 year old Angela Zhang who attends Monta Vista High School in California. She started developing a cure for cancer when she was 15. Angela had an idea to mix cancer medicine in a polymer that would attach to nanoparticles that would then attach to cancer cells, which would show up on an MRI. She then aimed infrared light at the tumors to melt the polymer and release the cancer medicine. This proved to kill cancer cells while leaving healthy cells unharmed. And what about "researchers in Canada"?

Researchers at the University of Alberta in Canada discovered a simple, inexpensive drug that is proven to kill cancer cells. The drug is called dichloroacetate (DCA). DCA changes the metabolism of cancer cells and causes them to age and die; a feat that is alien to cancer cells and stops them from otherwise destroying the human body. This drug has been around for quite some time and was proven to kill cancer cells in 2007. But it has been held up with a lot of testing and is not being funded very well.

This is going on with a drug that can very well bring an end to cancer.

So regardless of who has a cure for cancer or any disease, all cures are being ignored by the entire medical profession; even when a cure comes from one of their own.

But there's one thing I want to tell you about before I go on. It's about how radical I have been all these years in my knowledge of natural cures and medicines. But, I've also been right all long about natural healing and cures.

It wasn't too long ago that I happened to catch an episode of 60 Minutes on CBS. I saw them advertise that program and didn't want to watch it because I knew they would just say how stupid all of us are for saying anything bad about sugar and especially that sick crap known as high fructose corn syrup. But my wife and I sat and watched the show, knowing what they were gonna do. The only hope was that Dr. Sanjay Gupta was hosting the segment we wanted to watch. I kept the remote in my hand, ready to turn it, to keep from hearing their nonsense. But as it turns out, I got a big surprise from that segment.

Dr. Robert Lustig of the University of California at San Francisco is called a pioneer in what some call the war against sugar. The main diseases Dr. Lustig says are linked to sugar are type II Diabetes, Obesity, Hypertension and Heart disease. He says the American lifestyle is killing us and at least 75% of it is preventable. Dr. Lustig has published at least a dozen articles on the evils of sugar. But the way most people heard what he has to say is through his video on YouTube called Sugar: The Bitter Truth. Dr. Lustig and I are in agreement on everything except one point.

He says high fructose corn syrup is no worse than any other sugar. He does admit that it's the fructose that we crave, because there is fructose in every fruit; but not in the high amounts as in high fructose corn syrup. And in fruits that fructose is diluted by water, fiber and nutrients. That's why consuming fructose in fruits is the way to have a balanced diet. But when we consume high fructose corn syrup, it doesn't seem bad at all, since we were born to love fructose, in all our fruits, naturally.

In that same report, they told about a nutritional biologist at the University of California Davis who conducted a 5 year study linking excessive high fructose corn syrup consumption to diseases such as heart disease and stroke. Her study showed that calories from high fructose corn syrup effected the body differently than calories from other sources. She used a completely controlled environment in her study too.

Her subjects were in a kind of 24 hour lock down. Everything they ate was weighed and all calories were counted. They began eating normal meals, then began adding sugar in their diets so that 25% of their calories were from sugar. And in just two weeks, the ones who got 25% of their calories from high fructose corn syrup, had higher levels of bad cholesterol, LDL and other increased indicators of cardiovascular disease.

What they discovered was that when your liver gets overloaded with fructose, it begins converting it to fat, which produces LDL. That forms the plaque that clogs your arteries and blood vessels.

Their report also included some information on research studying the effects of sugar, glucose, on cancer cells. Cancer cells feed and grow by hijacking the flow of glucose in your blood stream. This is especially true with cancers known to have insulin receptors. And then there was the guy who did CAT scans on the brains of humans to see the effects of high fructose corn syrup on the brain.

He found out that high fructose corn syrup affects the brain in the same way as cocaine does. Dr. Sanjay Gupta volunteered to have CAT scans done while he was given a sip of soda pop through a tube. The CAT scan showed blood flow increased to certain parts of the brain as the soda hit his tongue. His brain began to release dopamine, as though it was some kind of addictive drug. The person conducting these tests on hundreds of people is Eric Stice, a Neuro Scientist at the Oregon Research Institute.

He concluded that as you eat more and more sugar, your body builds a tolerance to it. That causes you to crave more and more sugar as this tolerance level increases over time. This is exactly what happens when you are addicted to drugs. And that brings me to the surprise part of that segment. Actually it was the part that almost shocked me. I never thought I'd hear anyone BUT me say what I was about to hear from Dr. Lustig!

At one point, Dr. Sanjay Gupta is talking to this Dr. Lustig, the guy they said was leading the war on sugar, and Sanjay asks Dr. Lustig if he is going to go out on a limb and say that sugar is a toxin, a poison. Well, Dr. Lustig said he believes it is. But what about ME? I didn't go out on a limb recently and say sugar is a poison. No, that was Dr. Lustig.

I'm the guy who not only went out on a limb and said sugar is a poison. I said white granulated sugar is a drug. I didn't go out on a limb saying that. I rode a rocket ship off THAT limb. And I rode a rocket ship off that limb back at least 30 years ago; about 1981. So I was really thrilled to see this doctor and these scientists presenting solid scientific evidence to back up what I began saying 30 years ago. And in that segment, they also let one of those guilt ridden sugar cane farmers TRY to defend his crappy poisons.

Now, let's get this straight from the beginning. This sugar cane farmer could have just said that he grows the sugar cane. And it's not his fault that corporations take his natural sugar cane and make the drug called white granulated sugar, instead of making pure cane sugar. But he actually tried to defend this crap. And this is the pathetic destructive mentality that develops when all anyone cares about is money.

His sugar cane is good. Taking it and making drugs from it is what is wrong, wrong, wrong, wrong, wrong! But even though I appreciated that fine segment from CBS 60 Minutes, I had an alarmingly negative experience with one of their employees, former Miss America Debbye Turner.

Debbye grew up in the same city I did. Her grandmother lived across the street from us, and remained our neighbor when we moved a block away from her. So Debbye and I were "Friends" on FB. I had spoken to her in person before. But she is younger than me. So I didn't know her very well. One day Debbye makes a post on Facebook about a CBS news story she was doing about looking for a cure for cancer. So I commented on her post and gave her the cure for cancer. It was actually an abbreviated explanation and I also mentioned the cure was in my book Self-Care Health Care Guide.

I also offered it for free to all my Facebook friends and their FB friends. But after a couple of hours, no one had said anything in response to my comments. I couldn't find my comments. So I made another post asking Debbye why she deleted my comments. And her reply even shocked me. I can tell you plenty of things I have witnessed that would shock almost everyone. And only a tiny bit of that really shocks me.

Debbye said she was not going to tolerate hate speech from anybody. And before I could ask her what she was talking about, Debbye went ahead and said she was talking about me posting the cure for cancer on her post! As ridiculous as that was, I could only believe she was joking at that moment. But she kept on with that, and even got a couple of people to support her on her bold statement that posting the cure for cancer is "hate speech".

But that time with Debbye Turner was not the only time the haters have lashed out at me for saying there is a cure for cancer. But why did I share this with you? What good does it do to tell me all of this, you might ask. It's to give you some proof of how even the most well-respected people in this country are opposed to all cures and don't want anyone to know about cures, since cures take lots of money away from corporations.

I want you to cure yourself while you listen to your doctors, so you don't get all scared a lot of the time while you wait for your cure to become obvious. I wish I could tell you that your doctors, family and friends will support you in your efforts to cure yourself, but it's just not what I am able to tell you. Everyone will tell you to only listen to your doctors. And it won't matter that the doctors sentenced you to death. And it won't matter that without a cure, you are dead!

Thinking outside that tiny bubble about your health that doctors created over the past 75-100 years, is not something you are going to find support for. Even when you are advised to talk to your doctor before taking any herbal medications, they know that only a rare few doctors will say anything true or positive about anything that they don't make money off of. If doctors could patent Vitamin C, they would have gladly told you that Vitamin C cures the common cold. But since no one has a patent on Vitamin C, we're told there IS no cure for the common cold.

But no matter how hard doctors and the medical profession and drug companies ignore natural substances in favor of their artificial substitutes for most all natural substances, you still need a cure for your cancer. And that is THE most important thing. So DO what I laid out in this book. And use chapters 5, 6 and 7 as a daily guide to eliminate or at least greatly reduce the amount of poisons going into your body. Your health will change for the better. Those changes for the better will become noticeable within a few weeks. And as those changes in your health for the better continue to increase over the next months, your goal of curing yourself of cancer will become a reality to you.

The cure for cancer is not really a secret. I have seen plenty of cases of people curing themselves of cancer on the VERIA TV network. There were several people with stage 4 cancer who cured themselves doing an important part of what I tell you to do in this book; which is making the effort to change to what I call The Perfect Diet. One woman I remember, had just a few months to live and was also pregnant. And she is still telling her story here 30 years later. She gave birth to a son too. She turned a horrible horrible situation into the most wonderful event in her life, by believing she COULD be cured and dwelling on natural things instead of the artificial means provided by this nation's medical profession.

So let me remind you one more time about WHAT a cure is. **A cure is the thing that saves you from sickness and gives you Life instead of Death.** In my world, cures are second only to family and other living things in importance. If I had rode the pony the doctors gave me to ride, I would be dead; and there would be no books from me to help anyone. So cures are HUGE in my world. I have come to realize that even though cures have been ignored by the general Public over the past 75 years ,that more and more people just want to be cured.

And since doctors have no cures, you are only going to find out about these cures from someone like me. You can also check historical facts, like reading up on Hippocrates, the Father of Medicine. Then you will know doctors do NOTHING Hippocrates did. But it's all good news to everyone BUT the medical profession. No one but them stopped them from doing as Hippocrates.

About half of what I told you in this book closely resembles holistic medicine.

That's because the cure for cancer and all disease deals with your whole body problem. Your cancer doesn't come by itself. No disease comes by itself. So treating symptoms is only good for prolonging your disease and running up all those medical bills that bankrupt a million Americans each year. But the most important facts for being cured are not taught in holistic medicine. And that is the part about the poisons that cause all disease, except for the 20% caused by germs and viruses. I saturated my kidneys with poisons that no one BUT me had ever called poisons. And I did so to the point that my kidneys turned to mush and failed, with my blood pressure going sky high to 240/140 for several months. All due to the fact that your liver converts excess high fructose corn syrup and other sugars to fats that become LDL in your blood stream.

There are cures for every disease. But they're all outside the medical profession. And when it comes to cancer, no doctor is gonna turn his back on all that money those chemotherapy drugs make them in favor of telling you that poisons caused your cancer, so you can do something about that problem.

But that's actually perfect with me. Why? Because I am a pure American. So I know the U.S. Constitution does two main things. One is to establish Individual Rights as the Supreme Authority of America. And even in the bible, Christ Jesus died so that each Individual could receive all that GOD has for you (His Holy Spirit) without any connection to any group, religion or christian church.

And when it comes to any possibility of you being cured, yes sir, yes mam! It's YOU, the Individual, that can save your own life, the lives of your loved ones; cure yourselves and make cures a part of your Life again. I cannot cure you and no doctor can cure you. YOU can cure YOU! That is so wonderful and Powerful and even more so when you compare that to the hopelessness of the helpless medical profession. But continue looking for any signs of progress toward cures. I believe the days of doctors being trusted like gods are over.

If you search for a cure, you will find it. And you have found the cure you were looking for right here. You can cure yourself WHILE you still listen to your doctors, except about death and there being no cure. And you can do it for very little money. And best of all, it all depends on YOU.

This book contains the knowledge to empower YOU to cure yourself. You must DO what this book says. And the more you do what this book says to do, the faster you will get positive results and those results will be more and more significant as you do more and more of what this book teaches you to do.

The point you want to get to is when you have learned to buy groceries and have read the labels on every product so many times that you only bring home a tiny bit of poisonous crap; or you have made the decision to leave the crap alone altogether. And you have gotten use to drinking your pure clean water as an essential habit to maintain good health. These are the lifestyle changes you are going to have to make. And I don't mean you have to give up your life. I mean that now you know that all the food in restaurants are bad for you, are you going to stop eating out as much as you have and only do so rarely? Or you just gonna keep on like you have been, down the path that led to you getting cancer and every disease you have.

I get kinda of skiddish when friends suggest I come over and eat with them. It's like my high school class reunions. There's no way I would eat the crap food you eat! All smoked red meats except for some chicken wings is what I see as the stupidity of willful ignorance, in relevance to eating healthy.

So you are going to have to make those lifestyle changes to sustain your cure and good health once it is restored. But while you work on that, make sure you focus on avoiding the poisons that saturate our entire food, drinks and water supplies. Because those poisons are the cause of your diseases.

I would wish you luck with doing what my book says. But it's all science. You don't need luck with science. You just use the science as it is. And that's what this book is about - the proven science about what causes all disease and how to recognize those poisons so you can avoid them and all the chronic diseases that they cause.

And last of all...... If you think you can really trust your doctor, who is supposed to BE a Physician by definition yet cures no one, just remember what doctors did back a few decades ago. Doctors were on TV not only assuring the Public that cigarettes are not bad for them, but that smoking cigarettes had various health "benefits". Then maybe you can get on over that hump of believing in death sayeth the doctors and getting on with curing yourself because that's what you want. That's what your family wants for you. And a cure is the only thing that is going to save your life.

I wish all of you the very best in your efforts and congratulate you on what you are about to discover; something that doctors say does not exist.....the cure for cancer and the world where that cure and all cures come from. It's the world you lived in as a child, but turned your back on once you got all grown up and didn't have to listen to anybody and nobody could tell you what to do any more.

And now it's time to be a child again and allow the power of knowledge to heal you and set you free of that world of hopelessness cancer and all disease brings to us and afflicts us with so horribly.

And may this saving knowledge reach all your loved ones and reach around the world to open the eyes of all who seek a cure for their cancer and other chronic diseases. Cures are here to stay. Embrace them and hold on to them as an important part of Life. Be safe. Be well.

11 - How to Avoid dialysis and Cure Chronic Kidney Disease

I wanted to cover another major disease that afflicts and eventually kills almost everyone who gets it. It's the disease I had to cure myself of to save my own life and forced me to discover the cure for all chronic disease. If you have kidney disease, you are about to embark on saving your own life and significantly improving your health and avoiding dialysis; on your way to most likely curing yourself. In this book you will find the information you need to do all of this. I will tell how you can avoid dialysis by contacting the only Doctor in the country that has helped over a thousand people to avoid dialysis through his drug treatments, which have been clinically proven to work.

And for those who wish to take responsibility for their own health and for those who prefer natural cures over drug treatments, I give you the complete story and details about how I became the first person in America to reverse my chronic kidney disease and cure myself. And what I did, not only cured my chronic kidney disease, but cured me of every disease and medical condition I had. I cured myself of 20+ years of arthritis, intestinal bleeding, bleeding gums, headaches and heartburn.

I also cured myself of an enlarged heart and gout; as well as pulling myself back from the brink of diabetes. But my first experience with curing chronic "incurable" disease was in 1996 when I cured myself of "incurable" bladder stones after four excruciatingly painful attacks in just 3 or 4 years. I did so without doctors, by taking Magnesium oxide and Vitamin C.

As a matter of fact, I cured myself after stopping my fourth bladder stone attack WHILE it was in progress! I took 2 400mg Magnesium oxide tablets about an hour after the fourth attack started. And within 45 minutes, the attack began to fade away. And that was the end of it. No one was more shocked than I was. I have kept taking Magnesium since then to insure I would not have any more bladder stones or develop kidney stones or bone spurs. And I did it with proven science which doctors refuse to be interested in.

So I am shoutin' from the roof tops about what I did, so that chronic kidney disease and all disease can be brought to an end, or at least a bare minimum. I celebrate still being alive every day by talking about what cured me. And what cured me is written in this book for you to follow and cure yourself. I can only tell you that you WILL cure yourself, because that is the only way I know. But since I do not know all the different situations people face in having kidney disease, some MAY not be cured. But the least you will achieve is significantly improving your health and adding days, weeks and years to your life. And that's something you can't get from doctors.

If you want a doctor that will use clinically proven drug treatments to arrest your kidney disease so you don't have to go on the dialysis machine, you can contact Dr. Moskowitz to participate in his drug treatments. That will enable you to avoid dialysis and put your chronic kidney disease in check. But even though Dr. Moskowitz's drug treatments have been proven in clinical trials and that data given to the National Institute of Health, they have refused to do their basic duty of sending that information out to the medical profession. You would think they would be interested in saving lives and saving some of that $50 billion a year that the government spends on dialysis and Medicare and Medicaid payments for patients with chronic kidney disease.

But they aren't interested in the least bit. And they have refused to get the data from Dr. Moskowitz to the medical community. But these cold hearted monsters are not alone in this gruesome behavior!

Just go to www.GenoMed.com for more information. He has proven drug treatments for other diseases besides chronic kidney disease too. Dr. Moskowitz is just one of the two doctors that has helped me at all. It's just that his drug treatments do not cure you. They only stop your kidney disease from getting worse. That keeps you off dialysis and you get better as long as you stay on the drug treatments. There are no adverse effects that take place with Dr. Moskowitz's proven drug treatments. He uses a specific blood pressure medicine in high doses to achieve his stated results.

Low doses of this drug control the side of the gene that causes high blood pressure associated with kidney disease and high doses control and arrest the other side of the gene causing your kidney disease; as I understand it and also experienced it.

When I was searching the INTERNET to begin writing this book, I did a Google search for avoiding dialysis to see if anyone had finally written a book about avoiding dialysis or curing chronic kidney disease. And whose web site came up almost at the top? A site/company called Davita. I clicked the link and it took me to a forum discussion board for kidney patients.

I couldn't find anything about avoiding dialysis on their site forum. So I started a topic about me curing myself of chronic kidney disease. But as posters began to attack and ridicule me for this, I began to question whether that site had anything to do with helping kidney patients. As I backed up on the URL and go to the root/home page of that forum, it turned out to be a company that provides dialysis services for kidney patients. And it was no surprise when this heartless, immoral dialysis company banned me from their site permanently just 3 days later!

The vicious intolerance of cures by the entire medical profession is an ugly but real thing. But let's not pick on heartless Davita.com. Heck, I sent emails with detailed information to the National Kidney Foundation about me reversing and curing myself of chronic kidney disease. And I haven't heard one little peep from them; not even a congratulations on being cured from them! All these hypocrites are just support for the failed medical profession. They are of no value to anyone who wishes to get better or be cured! But my first experience with this vicious heartless attitude of doctors and the medical profession came from my own doctors. And it only took them about 18 months to show me they are intolerable of anyone getting better or curing themselves.

The doctors that diagnosed me with chronic kidney disease ended up throwing me out of their clinic, refusing to be my doctors any more. Once they saw me improve on my own without any help from them for my kidneys, they sent me certified letters stating they would no longer be my doctors.

I kept those letters in case they claim this is not true. I started off with those doctors and clinic with my Creatinine at 2.9 and climbing to 3.1 two months later; on course for the 0.1 monthly rise in Creatinine that leads all kidney patients to the dialysis machine. Those doctors got their first proof that I was doing what they had never done when my lab results came back 5 months later and my Creatinine was down to 2.6.

Then when my lab tests came back 11 months after that and my Creatinine was down to 2.2, they knew I was curing myself or at least reversing my kidney disease with a sustained remission. Barely six weeks later, I get those certified letters stating that my 2 doctors would no longer be my doctors.

It was during the next months following me receiving those certified letters that I found Dr. Moskowitz's GenoMed site and contacted him. So because of that, I was so glad those worthless doctors of Death and dialysis did me a favor by kicking me out of their clinic and refusing to be my doctors. I have mentioned Dr. Moskowitz in other places in this book. Dr. Moskowitz's drug treatments work if you want all the help you can get NOW. I used Dr. Moskowitz's drug treatments until the end of 2011. And would return to them if there is ever any indication I am developing kidney disease again.

If you have the printed version of this book or a PDF version, then you can check the Index for Dr. Moskowitz. But why did I tell you this about doctors and the medical profession?

I did it for a few reasons. First, it's no secret that there is no cure for chronic kidney disease in the medical profession. So if you want to be cured, then doctors and the medical profession are not of any value with that, because doctors never studied cures in Medical school. So they can't cure you and don't even have any interest in curing you. You need the medical profession to do what they actually do – take tests and diagnostics and prescribe drugs. If you are going to cure yourself or improve your health that is something you are going to have to do on your own. And to do that, you must empower yourself with the knowledge that will cure you or at least greatly improve your health.

That fact excites me every time I think about it! You have no hope. There is no cure. Doctors can't do a thing to help your kidneys get better. In just a very short time you will be on the dialysis machine as you wait for a possible kidney transplant that may or may not work. And as the symptoms slowly increase and progress, you must decide when dialysis could be better than continuing to suffer with all the symptoms you have. And until Dr. Moskowitz started helping people avoid dialysis for years, the only help kidney patients had was Dr. Mackenzie Walser's book Coping With Kidney Disease – A 12 Step Program to Help You Avoid Dialysis; which was to learn Dr. Walser's low 20 gram daily protein diet to arrest the progression of chronic kidney disease.

That is all the help I ever found in all the hours I spent trying to find anything that might or would help my kidneys. And I know just about all of you with chronic kidney disease are going through these same difficulties and hopelessness from doctors and the medical profession. You don't have the time to waste with being mad at doctors or trusting them. You are going to die very soon unless YOU do something about it.

Most people have told me that "God gave you the sense to know to go to the doctor." But I tell them that's the problem. Your "God" didn't give you the sense to know to go to the doctor and get a cure, OR LOOK ELSEWHERE until you find a cure!!!!!" And that is the beginning of the attitude changes you have to make in order to cure yourself. And since poisons in our food, drinks and water supplies cause all disease, you can learn to avoid those poisons that caused your disease and cure yourself on your own. And you can do it WHILE you still go to your doctors who have no cures. Another attitude you must change is about cures.

Your present attitude about cures is that there is no cure. There are no cures. But how about facing the fact that there is a cure for every disease known to man, but they're all OUTISIDE the medical profession. But the great thing is that you can afford the cures. What you cannot afford is the treatments for your disease as you are led down the path to dialysis and Death. And dialysis costs $100,000 a year per patient.

So start changing your way of thinking and remember that there is a cure for every disease. You just have to take the time to find it. This chapter focuses on the millions of people with the same disease I cured myself of. But no matter what disease you have, doing what chapters 5, 6 and 7 tell you to do will improve your health and most likely cure you of any disease you have. And that means all the diseases doctors pretend are "incurable". Make cures a part of your daily thinking and work to make cures a part of your life and the lives of your family and other loved ones.

So, you **train yourself to remember there is a cure for every disease known to man. And you look for those cures until you find them. And you keep cures as a part of your life from now on! You know what a CURE is? A CURE is the thing that saves your life from sickness and disease.**

But when it comes to the United States, the key to curing yourself of any and all disease is by reducing and eventually eliminating as much of the poisons you consume through food, drinks and unfiltered water, as you possibly can. And that's what this book is mainly about. But you'll need at least one more attitude adjustment to see these facts clearly. That's because you actually trust the FDA.

Yes, it's the FDA that says all these disease causing, addicting poisons are "safe". The FDA is also the ones who claim those prescription drugs that kill at least 25,000 Americans each year are "safe". The FDA claims all these poisons are "safe" as long as they don't kill you right away. You already know your parents told you poisons are harmful! But you forgot that because the FDA says poisons are safe as long as they're in your food, drinks and water. The solution is simple. Stop believing that poisons are safe. Start learning what these poisons are. Find them in your food and drinks and wherever they are and avoid them. But be warned – once you start doing this, the grocery store gets smaller and smaller. I mean tiny!

I can only think about how excited I am for all of you who are about to get started doing what this book says to do and save your lives and add so much more time to your lives. Oh how I WISH I had this book to help me when I was dying, on the road to dialysis in just months. So I am so thrilled to provide for all of you the information I needed to save my life, avoid dialysis and become the first person in this country to cure myself of chronic kidney disease. And lucky for you, I did not include hardly anything that did NOT work (except for doctors and the medical profession).

I will tell you up front that much of this book is taken from an earlier book of mine titled Self-Care Health Care Guide. I could just about take chapters 5, 6 & 7 and build a book for each and every disease around those chapters. This is due to the huge fact that poisons cause all disease except the 20% caused by germs and viruses. The fact that all of us need help in cleaning up our current diets is the entire reason behind the information in those chapters. It's either follow those chapters OR simply become a vegetarian.

Please feel free to write us and tell us your story about how you cured yourself or greatly improved your health or about you avoiding dialysis because of what you read and learned in this book.

If you want to reduce the number of pages you read and still get all the help you need, just skip chapter 12. That chapter is just about my experiences I had with the medical profession after developing CKD. Such a tiny trickle of help came from all that time and money spent with them. I only included the next chapter to give you the details of my experiences with doctors and the modern medical profession as I went to them for a cure and help in getting better, but got either! It's not essential to your cure. But there are a few great tips in chapter 12.

You're Probably Dying, So Let's Get You Some Help

Let me say this very clearly and as strongly as I can. **This book has NO GIMMICKS. This book presents scientific facts that give the results stated in this book. It is up to YOU to take these scientific facts about your body, disease and the food, drinks and water you consume and put that science to work for you, to train and force your body to heal itself naturally.**

Basically, you learn to recognize the saturation of poisons in your food, drinks and water, in order to avoid, reduce and eliminate those poisons. You should drink plenty of pure clean water. Correct your major nutrient deficiencies. And fast as often as possible to speed your healing along. A fast of 12-16 hours is easy to achieve on a regular basis

If you got this book, then you are probably dying right now. So you need to get right to the facts that are going to keep you off dialysis and cure your chronic kidney disease. I know I searched many many hours and days for any little shred of information that might help my kidneys get better. But there is little information in the world that can help you. The main reason is because no one has had any success in helping kidney patients get better or cured.

You went to the doctor and he told you that you have kidney disease and that there is no cure for it. They tell you that you will progressively get worse and eventually die from your kidney disease. And that all they can do is help you with the symptoms of chronic kidney disease as they develop.

The typical story for a kidney patient is that they first have elevated levels of Creatinine and BUN in their blood. But the first sign of trouble is usually a problem with Potassium (K). Your muscles will become tight and give you cramps if you're low on Potassium. And if your Potassium is too high, you will experience heart palpitations which are life threatening. Your heart pounds out of control. If your blood pressure is high, you will bruise easily.

As your Creatinine rises at the rate of 0.1 each month, you began to get swelling in your ankles and face from the water not being properly controlled. Your skin begins to itch more and more. And by the time your Creatinine reaches 5.0+ 2-3 years after getting chronic kidney disease, you have to decide WHEN you want to start dialysis.

One thing you have to decide is who you are going to listen to? **Are you going to continue listening to the doctors who have no cures and won't do anything to help your kidneys get better? OR, you going to listen to someone like me who did what no doctors have ever done and cured myself of chronic kidney disease?**

The first book I wrote about this is called Self-Care Health Care Guide. But I didn't restrict the information in that book to just curing chronic kidney disease. That's because the cure for chronic kidney disease is also the basic cure for almost all disease. I am writing this part of the book to concentrate on the 30

Million Americans that have chronic kidney disease and anyone and everyone else in the world that has this always fatal disease.

You don't realize the value of your kidneys until you get kidney disease. Then you don't understand what is happening to you. I want to talk about that right now, but later I will go into exactly what happened to me as I hopelessly tried to get the medical profession to help my kidneys get better. The doctors even made remarks on my medical records implying that I am crazy because I kept asking them what they were going to do to help my kidneys and I kept telling them I was going to be cured. But I was crazy because I thought THEY were going to cure me. I didn't know that doctors have no cures until I went to the doctors for cures in 2006. So the medical profession is a two-edged sword.

You naturally turn to the medical profession to find out what is wrong with you after you get sick and habitually feel bad. **The medical profession is very helpful in diagnosing diseases. They are the exclusive source for prescription drugs, lab tests, surgeries, treatments for sickness and medical procedures. But the things that they can't help you with are cures and medicine. They don't teach cures in their medical schools, so doctors never learn the cures that have been around for many centuries.**

All the medicines man had were herbs. Herbs are merely plants that have been used as medicines. That classifies and defines them as herbs.

But yet no doctors in the modern medical profession has studied medicine; herbs. My doctor told me outright that he didn't know a thing about herbs (medicine). And it doesn't matter to any doctors that they swore an oath to Hippocrates, the Father of Medicine, whose practice was founded on herbs and fasting. But I am not telling you to do without doctors. I am clarifying what doctors CAN and CAN NOT do for you.

You will need some of their drugs for high blood pressure and maybe a thing or two besides. And you will need them to test your blood to see how well your cure is coming along and that your Creatinine level is no longer increasing. You may want to get an Ultrasound if you are paying cash and a CT Scan if your insurance will pay for it.

But the first thing your doctor will do if you seem to have kidney problems is determine whether or not your kidney problems are being caused by kidney stones. **So before I give you the information on How to Avoid Dialysis and Cure (chronic) Kidney Disease, let's see if your kidney problems are caused by kidney stones. Then I'll give you the cure for kidney stones.**

What If My Kidney problem is Kidney stones?

The first thing doctors will look into if there is a problem with your kidneys found in your blood tests, is to see if you have kidney stones. If you have kidney stones, you can either dissolve them naturally or have them surgically removed.

Kidney stones are cured the same way bladder stones and bone spurs are cured. The one factor that makes kidney stones different is the effect of uric acid in forming uric acid kidney stones. Over production of Uric acid is what causes gout. But its role in forming kidney stones is what separates the cure for uric acid kidney stones from calcium based kidney stones, bladder stones and bone spurs. Drinking lots of water and baking soda water is the basic cure for Uric Acid stones, while Magnesium is the cure for calcium based kidney stones.

Too much Uric acid for prolonged periods of time leads to uric acid stones. Uric acid is produced when purines break up. Purines are found in foods like meat, peas, beans, liver and some alcoholic drinks. So avoid a diet high in animal protein. It is very important to drink a lot of water to help prevent and cure any kidney stones. You can't allow excess uric crystals to remain in the kidneys and form these uric acid stones. Drinking 2-3 quarts of pure water a day will help pass around 90% of kidney stones. So don't forget! Adding pH drops to the water and drinking baking soda and water is even better.

And don't forget the magnesium, if you have calcium kidney stones, which will dissolve this most common type of kidney stones. B6 also acts like Magnesium in the body. The science this cure comes from is that Magnesium is needed in the body to dissolve calcium so that calcium can be used by your body. If you don't have enough magnesium, these undissolved calcium particles are free to bind to toxins(free radicals, poisons) to form stones in your kidneys, as well as in your bladder. You need antioxidants such as Vitamins C, A & E, as well as lesser known antioxidants like Selenium and Alpha Lipoic Acid and others to remove toxins from your body. You need the Magnesium to dissolve calcium. This one-two punch of vitamin supplementation can cure you of calcium based kidney and bladder stones and bone spurs.

To cure yourself of calcium based kidney stones, you need to take at least 800mg Magnesium oxide and 3000-5000mg Vitamin C daily until cured. The stones will dissolve slowly over a short period of time because of the excess magnesium; perhaps 6-8 weeks, or longer if the stones are bigger than usual.

And by taking the Magnesium oxide, over 300 body metabolisms will begin occurring in your body after years of no activity; due to the Magnesium deficiency in your diet all these years. Vitamin supplementation is not a gimmick. It's an essential requirement for your health, due to our parched, lifeless, hallow food supply. Just ask yourself WHERE are you getting your daily supply of Magnesium in your food? Yea, I know. You can't tell me or yourself!

Now the way you can almost always determine for yourself whether you have kidney disease or whether you have calcium kidney stones or uric acid stones is by doing this:

You almost always notice any kidney problems by the back ache you will get in your lower back. It's not pain. It's aching as though you are just having lower back muscle problems. If you have kidney disease or calcium kidney stones, your lower back will ache almost all the time, BUT, you won't have sharp pains. If your back pain includes sharp pains frequently, then you most likely have uric acid stones. But before I tell you the cure for uric acid kidney stones, I need to explain what to do to determine if your problem is developing chronic kidney disease or calcium kidney stones. Determining this is simple, but takes time.

Merely follow my previous instructions to dissolve any calcium kidney stones. And at the same time, drink the baking soda water 3-4x daily in case you have Uric Acid stones. If you don't improve within 5-6 weeks, then you most likely have chronic kidney disease. **But my strongest advice is to do this, AND start eliminating the saturation of poisons in your food, drinks and water supplies to significantly improve your overall health and speed your cure and natural healing along.** Use chapters 5, 6 and 7 for guiding you in eliminating the saturation of poisons in our food, drinks and water supplies; most of which we all pretend are food!

Uric Acid kidney stones – You most likely have uric acid stones from too much uric acid formation from consuming high fructose corn syrup. These stones cannot be cured the same way calcium based kidney stones are cured. To cure uric acid stones drink baking soda and water. You must read food and drinks labels and avoid high fructose corn syrup; especially in liquid forms such as soda pops and fruit juice too. Doing so will decrease your body's production of uric acid. The other part of the cure for uric acid stones is to drink lots of pure water to dissolve and flush these stones out of your body.

The suggested amount of water is 1-ounce for every 2 pounds of body weight daily. Your kidneys love water. But it needs to be filtered to remove the harmful chlorine and fluoride in the water. Add pH drops or baking soda too.

A carbon water filter only filters out about 90% of the chlorine and nothing else. So that's why you need a fluoride water filter at least. A reverse osmosis is better and filters all your water in your home. Using either of these water filters takes all the taste out of your water that you taste in tap water. The chemicals are bitter and acidic. So by removing chlorine and fluoride, the bitter acidic taste is gone. Then your water is alkaline. The easiest way to increase the alkalinity of your water is to add baking soda or pH drops to your drinking water every day. This raises the pH to around 7.5-8.0 and above.

Flushing your kidneys with this highly alkaline water will neutralize acid and slowly transform your body's acidic state back into the normal alkaline state your body is suppose to be in. Your body became acidic over time as you consumed more and more animal products, sugar and chlorinated water. And the highly alkaline water reverses that disease ripe acidic environment inside your body. Chlorine destroys the oxygen in every cell it comes into contact with and kills the beneficial bacteria in your stomach and intestines.

One side effect of the highly alkaline water will be weight loss. As the highly alkaline water neutralizes acid in your body, your kidneys will remove all that water it retained to dilute that acid, as a natural defense to that acid. That is how you lose the weight.

But if none of this causes your lower back ache to go away, you most likely have chronic kidney disease. If so, you will want to read on for the information that will help you and most likely cure you. You can contact Dr. David Moskowitz to participate in his drug treatments to put your kidney disease in check. But before I get to the cure and how to avoid dialysis naturally, let me tell you what the doctors did to determine if I had kidney stones.

Well actually they did nothing. But what they wanted me to do and insisted I do was get some CAT scans of my kidney area at St. Bernard's hospital. When the doctor told me this I said "Why? There's no way I could have kidney stones because I take magnesium." Him and the nurse looked at me like what the heck is he talking about. (Sad, but true, since it's proven medical science.)

I asked the employees who scheduled these tests about how much it would cost. No one could tell me. Even St. Bernard's couldn't tell them either until a day later. The cost was $1100. So there was no way I was paying cash for tests that expensive that contradict scientific facts. So I didn't take the CAT scans. Didn't throw away $1100 on tests that were proven to be unneeded tests.

No. I stuck with proven science instead of trusting the doctor's word that I needed those tests. I didn't have kidney stones and have never had kidney stones. I did have bladder stones in the mid-1990s. And after 4 immensely excruciatingly painful bladder stone attacks, I stopped my fourth bladder stone attack within an hour by talking 2 400mg Magnesium oxide tablets. I take Magnesium 3 or 4 times a week every week and haven't had another bladder stone since then, 1996. This was the first time I cured myself of what doctors call "chronic, incurable disease".

It doesn't matter if you have kidney stones, chronic kidney disease or any chronic disease. Doing what chapters 5, 6 & 7 tell you to do will significantly improve your health and most likely cure you of your chronic diseases. Chronic kidney disease is the deadliest disease, since 100% with chronic kidney disease die from it. Most develop diabetes and die from that. Some develop heart disease. And at some time, most of the rest will go on dialysis, while a small number will receive kidney transplants. Around 20,000 kidney transplants are performed in the United States each year. The waiting list for a transplant has 93,000 people on it and expands each year by 3000-4000 people.

And just as it is with cancer and any disease, an extremely important thing you should do is use an inexpensive, common substance known as baking soda. It reverses the acidic condition that allowed your kidney disease to survive and thrive in your body. Chronic disease can NOT live in an alkaline environment. Baking soda is also called meetha soda in some countries like Pakistan. Diseased cells are also more acidic than other cells in the body.

Baking soda is pH 14, and when mixed with water makes the entire glass of water become a pH of 8.0-8-5 and slightly higher if you use a carbon water filter, fluoride filter or an osmosis system. Merely mixing 1/2 tea spoon in 4-6 ounces of water and drinking twice daily, before bed and when you awake, will serve as the foundation for your near certain cure.

I finally cured my gout after I started drinking baking soda water and adding pH drops to my drinking water. It's all simple science. Gout is caused by Uric acid. Highly alkaline substances like baking soda and pH drops neutralize acid, thus reducing the acidic state of your body. It is acid that causes inflammation in your body. So by neutralizing Uric acid with baking soda water and pH drops, you cure your gout.

We use baking soda to neutralize acids, fungi and molds anywhere we find them. We also brush our teeth by wetting our brush and covering the brush with baking soda and brushing. We also brush some on our underarms as deodorant. You can also wet your fingers, dip them in the box of baking soda and rub it on your underarms for the best deodorant. We also used baking soda as a plant fungicide. Works great! So don't ever do without your baking soda!

The rest of this chapter is about what you can do to significantly improve your health and most likely cure yourself. And the key word there is YOU! I am going to tell YOU how to cure yourself of chronic kidney disease! I am also going to tell you how I cured myself of chronic kidney disease without any help from doctors, after doctors said I would be dead or on dialysis by late 2008 or early 2009. I started developing kidney disease in August 2005 and was diagnosed with chronic kidney disease in October 2006. My creatinine was 3.1 in December 2006.

I will give you the information to avoid dialysis and tell you how you can cure yourself and avoid dialysis by doing what I tell you in chapters 5, 6 & 7; along with other valuable information to help with your cure.

How to Cure Kidney Disease Naturally, Without Doctors

If you want to cure yourself or at least significantly improve your health, then I can tell you how to do that. That's what I had to do for myself to save my own life, after doctors said I would be dead or on dialysis by 2008. And even when you are on dialysis, it's almost like already being dead. I had one friend for sure that was just in his 30's when he started dialysis. He didn't last but 3 or 4 years after he started dialysis. And his quality of life was real bad too. So I was almost terrified as I looked to the future and knew I would soon be dead or on dialysis.

But no matter who I talked to, I never found any hope of anyone getting better once they had chronic kidney disease. I searched and searched the INTERNET for cures for kidney disease and avoiding dialysis from the day doctors told me I had chronic kidney disease. But I couldn't find anything. About the only help I found was a book by Dr. Mackenzie Walser called Coping with Kidney Disease: A 12-Step Program to Help You Avoid Dialysis.

Dr. Walser's book detailed his clinical research with his patients in testing his variation of a zero protein diet used by the British to successfully delay dialysis. Dr. Walser created a low protein diet to delay dialysis. The best this could do was to achieve what is called arrested progression. This means the progression of your chronic kidney disease has been arrested, stopped. But Dr. Walser states this is not remission. Remission is where you reverse the kidney disease and your kidneys improve for longer than a few months or you cure your kidney disease. Well, I know Dr. Walser would be thrilled to know what I achieved.

But what are the details of that "cure"? First of all, I don't have any symptoms of chronic kidney disease any more. At first, my blood pressure was 240/140. I pissed blood and blood clots. I was excruciatingly tense and tight all over my body from low Potassium. I spent at least 2/3 of every day trying to piss, but barely did. I couldn't sleep but maybe 2 hours a night for weeks.

Then once I begin to get lab test results, my above normal results were Creatinine at 2.9 and my BUN was 30. I was also leaking protein into my urine. And my Potassium was below normal at 2.9. My EKG showed that I had an enlarged heart and I had dozens of bruises all over my body where blood vessels had popped from the 240/140 blood pressure. And when my next lab results came back, they showed I was getting worse! My Creatinine continued to climb to 3.1. My BUN jumped to 44. And my Potassium jumped from 2.9 to 5.7. Normal for those 3 are 1.5, 8-24 and a 3.5 - 5.0 range for Potassium.

But since I began doing the things I shared with you in chapters 5, 6 and 7, my Creatinine has been as low as 1.8. My Potassium has been normal the whole time. And everything else in my blood serum lab tests have been normal. My EKGs also changed and the results were good, then very good. I never have those attacks of shortness of breath that are caused by an enlarged heart. My doctor began treating me as though I am not a kidney patient. He has his own scientific proof of what I have done.

So whether you agree that I have cured myself, I know you can all agree that I sure live in the threshold of being cured. I have been there since the middle of 2007; even though I didn't realize I had actually succeeded in reversing my chronic kidney disease until I sustained that remission for a few years.

In 2009 I began to dismiss dialysis and Death as my only future and began to take my life back and start living again. In 2010, I was continuing to take my life back. And in 2011, I began to be a useful, productive person again. I wrote my first two books in 2011 and this is my 6th book since overcoming death and taking back my life and health. I have became more and more active, with the fear of dialysis and death having become just a faded memory behind me.

Dialysis is not the solution you want. It is very hard on you. It's a fact that 1 out of every 5 people who go on dialysis, take themselves off of dialysis; as death is a better choice than dialysis to that 20%. I for one, celebrate every day about how I am still alive and dialysis free, here in 2013; nearly eight years after my chronic kidney disease first began to develop and progress. My CKD began in August 2005. It took me almost 20 months after it began, to begin to arrest my kidney disease. And that still continues to this very moment.

So HOW did I manage to do what no doctors have ever done and do so without any real help from doctors? That is what I will be explaining now and giving you the information you need to empower yourself to cure yourself or at least significantly improving your health and extending your life by days, weeks and most likely for years. And you can do what I did, even if you participate in Dr. Moskowitz's drug treatments to avoid dialysis and even WHILE your doctors hold your hand and lead you to your grave as they prolong your illness to maximize their income.

You WILL become the doctors' $100,000 a year dialysis pony unless you contact Dr. Moskowitz, or do what I did, OR BOTH!

So here we go with my way and the ONLY way of reversing chronic kidney disease and avoiding dialysis naturally. What you have to do is change your diet. It's the saturation of poisons in our food, drinks and water supplies that are making us all sick to the point that over 130,000,000 Americans have at least one chronic disease. All disease is caused by poisons, toxins, chemicals; except for the 20% caused by germs and viruses. Your kidneys are the main organ for removing toxins from your body. And as you overload your kidneys with poisons, those poisons back up in your kidneys begin to become saturated with those poisons. Your kidneys begin to turn to mush, then your kidney disease becomes noticeable. But by then, it's too late.

When this happened to me, I not only had to deal with being sick, I had to figure out something that might help my kidneys get better. The doctors sure did nothing for my kidneys; even though I asked them to help my kidneys every time I went to the doctor! They even began to think I was crazy because I kept telling them I wanted to be cured. I didn't realize it while it was happening. I read it on my medical records later. I'm dying and they won't help! So what are you going to do?

Do everything this book says to do in chapters 5, 6 and 7. Chapter 5 is called Poisons in Your Water. I explain things about the water we drink; including bottled water. To sum the chapter up, simply forget about bottled water. PERIOD. And get a shower filter and a drinking water filter; preferably a fluoride filter. That's because a fluoride filter removes everything BUT the water at a rate of about 99%.

A shower filter is a special hot water filter that eliminates at least 90% of the chlorine in your shower water. Doing that cures dandruff and dry itchy red spots caused by the chlorine destroying the oils in our scalp and skin and kills the oxygen in every cell it comes into contact with. Without a shower filter, you are absorbing chlorine and fluoride through every pore on your body, while breathing chlorine gas in the steam of the hot shower water. So this is a major source of poisons for everyone. And that makes a shower filter a MUST for kidney patients.

Chapter 6 talks about the saturation of poisons in our drinks, like sodas, fruit juices and milk. Beware of how sad these facts are. It's rare to find any drink product at the grocery store that is NOT saturated with poisons. I do explain some alternatives which you can drink that aren't highly poisonous. But it pretty much comes down to Stevia sweetened tea, 2%, Skim and Organic milk. There is also a new soda, like 7-UP, called Sierra Mist.

Then in chapter 7, I give you the information to guide you in greatly reducing and eliminating almost all poisons from your food supply. It includes detailed information about sugars and also about the fraudulent labeling terms most food corporations use to try and trick you into buying their fake "healthy" products! You can't allow yourself to be fooled by terms like Natural, All Natural, Low Fat, Reduced Fat, Low Calorie, 100% Juice and other big fat lies. And there is no worse poison than high fructose corn syrup. It was high fructose corn syrup in the sodas and fruit juices I drank daily for about 5 years that are responsible for my kidney failure.

Now before I end this chapter so I can get on to the information that saved my life and reversed my chronic kidney disease, I need to explain some rules, laws, principles that my methods are founded on. If you take time to learn these scientific principles, you will value my methods much better and speed your cure along. It is these principles that my methods are founded on. One of those principles is about how your body can heal itself.

You have cut yourself before, right? Do you still have that cut? No. It healed on its own. And did you know that your liver can grow new cells. Say, if you had part of your liver removed, it grows back. So I am very confident in our bodies' ability to heal us of anything we do to ourselves, except for serious blunt trauma or the likes. You have to know how to make your body work to heal you better if you are going to cure yourself of chronic disease. One way to do that is to fast.

It is not necessary to fast for days. By simply eating your last meal around 6 PM, then not eating again until between 6 and 10 AM the next day, will do a lot for you; especially if you make it a habit. Fasting was the foundation of the medical practices of Hippocrates, the Father of Medicine. What fasting does is to relieve the body of the most energy consuming bodily task of digesting food.

Once your body ceases to digest food, your body then uses that energy to repair damaged cells in our bodies. And when you are sick, your body needs to use as much energy as possible to repair damaged cells and remove toxins, as it possibly can. And the less poisons you put into your body, the less energy your body has to use to remove those toxins. A good example is when you drink a soda pop.

People fool themselves by thinking that soda pop gives them a welcome energy boost! But it's no energy boost! What really happens is this:

You begin drinking that sugar soaked soda in liquid form with that DNA altering sodium benzoate and that 3.0 acidic carbonated water and your body goes into instant shock as it tries to defend itself against all that poison. This instant elevated activity the body goes into to remove these poisons is what we falsely tell ourselves is just an energy boost. And it takes your body up to 6 hours to remove the poisons in a 12-ounce soda pop. That cripples your immune system. And by drinking a 12-ounce soda every 6 hours, you in effect, nullify your immune system.

So, your body only has so much energy. It uses most of its energy to digest food. It uses the rest of its energy to remove toxins and repair damaged cells. So you have to learn how to make your body use more and more of its energy to repair damaged cells to heal and cure you. The easiest way to do that is to fast as often as possible and cut down on the amount of food you eat.

And as always - Use chapters 5, 6 and 7 to reduce the amount of poisons you consume in your food, drinks and water to relieve your body of having to use so much energy to remove toxins from your body. Doing this and fasting allows your body to use most of its energy to repair damaged cells; which eventually results in you being cured.

You also have to understand that you need to eat as healthy a diet and drinks as you can. I mean, why drink a soda or fruit juice when you could drink something that your body doesn't have to work so hard to remove all the poisons in that soda or juice. You could drink fruit smoothies made with raw fruits. That would be almost 100% good for your body. Those live fruits and vegetables have enzymes that pump life into your body. And your body doesn't work to remove that live produce. Your body uses most of that live produce. And if you juice that produce, it's easier for your body to digest than solid food.

It takes far less energy to digest that produce if you run them through a good juice making machine. But even if you don't juice or don't do it often, you can still try to eat as much raw fruits and vegetables as you possibly can.

As a matter of fact, if you just get those water filters and follow what I have been calling The Perfect Diet, you can cure yourself or significantly improve your health without having to learn how to read food labels and avoid the masses of products that are saturated with poisons; most of which we pretend are food. The Perfect Diet is the best diet to be on. But since it is a far cry from the "American diet", you may do best by using chapters 6 & 7 to clean up your current diet that caused your diseases in the first place.

More Help for Your Kidneys and Diabetes, Gout & Heart Disease

Everything I did the past five years was centered on my chronic kidney disease. I have tried all kinds of things. Most of them helped. A few did not help. The best thing for kidney disease is pure water. So start with a fluoride water filter as I pointed out in the Poisons in Your Water chapter. Drink 1-ounce of water for every 2 pounds of body weight. Drinking water is the best way to wash and cleanse your insides. But drinking water with chlorine and fluoride is almost enough to negate the positive effects water has on your kidneys and whole body. So at least get a carbon water filter to filter out 90% of the chlorine and no fluoride! They only cost $20-30.

Making sure you hold your blood pressure down is essential. Your doctor will tell you this. Take Hawthorn berries, L-Arginine, Fish oil, magnesium, B6 and garlic to help lower your blood pressure naturally, in addition to your prescribed medicines. Even Apple Cider Vinegar (ACV) can lower your blood pressure. It's high in vitamins that are helpful for lowering blood pressure, like Vitamins C, A, E, B1, B2 and B6, as well as Potassium, Magnesium and copper. ACV turns alkaline in the body which raises your body's pH levels. Valerian Root helps to calm you and lower blood pressure, but should be taken with caution and only according to directions. Dealing with stress goes a long way in controlling your blood pressure. So make sure you take measures to minimize your stress.

It is my opinion that you are best off taking Clonidine and Quinapril to control blood pressure artificially. Taking Atenolol only slows down your heartbeat to minimize the number of times your heart beats. But it doesn't actually lower your blood pressure. You could also take a CCB, Calcium Channel Blocker. But only do so for about a year at a time, since doing so any longer causes your PTH glands to release Calcium from your bones, which weakens them.

Due to the damage to your kidneys, which makes hormones to control your blood pressure, drugs to control blood pressure are almost always needed. This is the one area I am still working on to finish correcting. But I think it may take some artificial means of reversing the DNA or gene damage that caused this high blood pressure. I'm currently testing two other possibilities also.

The best thing I found to help my kidneys was a concentrated Chinese herbal product called Kidney Well. I always use Kidney Well and Alisma together. But you can get products from the same company for whatever your chronic kidney disease is. For their great kidney products visit their web site at: http://www.getwellnatural.com. I use Kidney Well as often as I can; which is at least every 3-6 months. It always helps. I usually take anywhere from 6-10 tablets of Kidney Well and 2-3 capsules of Alisma per dose 3 times daily on an empty stomach. It's good to take one of those doses right before bed time. There are no side effects to this herbal remedy, except for some light stomach discomfort occasionally. It gives you a clean feeling.

When it comes to holding down your protein, I have found that red meat is the hardest on your kidneys. So it was easy for me to get off red meat and just eat Omega-3 rich fish and chicken and turkey. You should take Bromelain with meals that include meat. Bromelain breaks down protein real well and is a natural product made from pineapple. Bromelain is also good at flushing excess protein out of your kidneys; a common problem for those with chronic kidney disease. Using Bromelain and papaya enzyme helps take the load off your pancreas in its role in digestion; which helps prevent diabetes.

Follow the instructions on page 72 to cure Diabetes, since Diabetes is the cause of 90% of kidney patients reaching end stage renal failure.

I drank gallons of Goji, Noni and Mangosteen Juice and ate Goji berries from time to time since first being diagnosed with chronic kidney disease. Regardless of any rumors of these being miracle cures, the extremely high anti-oxidant properties was reason enough for me to use these juices and berries. The problem is finding the rare few pure juices.

Stop cooking with the microwave. Only use the microwave oven to heat things, but only for 30 seconds or less. The damage cooking in a microwave does to food turns a good meal into a bad meal for your health. Microwaving food destroys up to 97% of the delicate vitamins and phytonutrients, plant medicines, in food.

If your doctor tries to trick you with white lies about your PTH hormone levels being high and you are on a Calcium channel blocker like Amlodipine, then simply ask your doctor to take you off the calcium channel blocker and switch it to an ACE inhibitor such as Quinapril, aka Accupril. Your Parathyroid glands control calcium levels in your body. Once your Parathyroid glands sense that the calcium channel blocker is blocking calcium to your heart, your Parathyroid glands will begin to release hormones, PTH. This causes your system to start releasing calcium from your bones into your blood stream to make up for that "simulated" calcium deficiency. Doctors only want you to do another drug to control the side effects of the first drug, the calcium channel blocker.

Avoid taking Ibuprofen, naproxen and aspirin. All of these are hard on your kidneys. If you work on avoiding poisons, the need for any of these over the counter drugs will become a thing of the past. Tylenol is hard on your liver. I have only taken 10 or 12 Aleve since mid-2007 and that was for severe tooth or back pain. And the last time I took any of those was around September 2010.

Your big problem is usually controlling your Potassium. Potassium is in just about everything you eat, but is highest in beans and peas; especially green beans. So don't eat beans or peas too often. 8-ounces of beans has as much Potassium as 3 or 4 oranges or bananas. Never eat more than 2 oranges or bananas in a day. One of each a day is as far as you should go. Cutting down on meat portions will help limit protein and Potassium too. Eating cheese and drinking milk and orange juice should be held to a minimum if you want to control your Potassium. 8-ounces of milk or orange juice contains around 300mg of Potassium, which is the same amount of Potassium in one medium orange or banana. One thing I have noticed is that even when I eat Potassium rich fruits, it doesn't seem to have the Potassium raising effect that meats have.

So lean toward eating fresh fruits and vegetables. I wish we could get watermelon year round. I am always thrilled to eat good watermelon. It is nothing but good for you. It is a great source of distilled water. A funny thing that is true is that if you really want the best detox program for your body, eat watermelon and soak in a hot tub as much as you can. Cantaloupe is great for the same reasons. You will notice how you have to pee more often after eating either one too. It's just proof of how much good it's really doing.

There aren't really any vitamins I take just for the kidneys. But I do take vitamins and herbs that do help my kidneys such as fish and flax seed oil, Taurine, Vitamin C, Vitamin E, B-Complex, L-Arginine, Astragalus and Bilberry. And the Kidney Well is a formula of about 5 herbs which includes Astragalus and Alisma. But make sure you steer clear of herbs like Licorice Root and Celery Seed. You can take Celery Seed as a diuretic as long as you are sure that your kidneys are not inflamed. Taking amino acids, B-Complex, will provide those B Vitamins you'll lose by restricting your protein consumption.

You can read Dr. Mackenzie Walser's book titled Coping With Kidney Disease: A 12-Step Program to Avoid Dialysis. His book gives you detailed information and instructions on restricting your protein intake. He kept lots of people off dialysis for years by putting his patients on protein restricted diets. He was a doctor and professor at John Hopkins Medical Center and University. His book was the only help I got from a doctor before I met Dr. Moskowitz.

As long as your creatinine isn't above 3.9, Dr. Moskowitz can probably keep you off dialysis. And even if your creatinine is above 3.9, he is still willing to try and help you. **Between his treatment and what I did to help my kidneys, as told in this book, I do not know of a single other thing that can help anyone with chronic kidney disease.** But hey...the entire medical profession can't and does not do a thing to help the kidneys of chronic kidney disease patients. They only treat the symptoms of CKD while they hold your hand and lead you to the dialysis machine and the grave.

(The following information is also available in chapter 8.)

Other diseases that are common among people with kidney disease are:

Gout - Gout is an extremely painful condition. Gout is caused by an overproduction and over population of uric acid. Uric acid has needle-like points on the crystals. The pain of gout is caused by those needle-like crystals. Just imagine tens of thousands of needles inside your big toe or ankle and you get the idea behind what gout is doing to you. Although most gout attacks are the result of consumption of high fructose corn syrup, especially in liquid form such as fruit juices and soda pops, gout is also caused by other things. The common factor among all the causes is the introduction of poisons or some other body trauma such as chemotherapy, joint injury and dehydration.

This tells you that drinking lots of pure water will help gout. And working on avoiding poisons in your food and drinks will cure your gout and/or prevent gout altogether. Drinking too much alcohol can bring on a gout attack. Alcohol is mostly a sugar and a poison to your body. Drinking beer and eating shrimp together are known to cause gout.

I cured myself of gout by getting off the high fructose corn syrup. And I nailed this fact down forever. I went through a phase for 2 to 3 months where I was tired of being laughed at and hated on because of my speaking out against high fructose corn syrup. So, I just gave it up and decided that since I'm so crazy for speaking out against high fructose corn syrup that I would now shut my crazy mouth and never do it again. And since, according to most everyone else, high fructose corn syrup is only a poison in MY crazy opinion, then it was perfectly safe for me to consume high fructose corn syrup.

I stopped trying to avoid high fructose corn syrup for 2-3 months. Then I got gout and had gout all day every day for two whole months! And that is what broke me and stood me up against high fructose corn syrup FOREVER! I mean this one is nailed down! But, to test this "opinion" of mine one final time, I told myself I would stay off the high fructose corn syrup, UNLESS I had another gout attack AFTER getting off the high fructose corn syrup again.

But you really need to work on avoiding poisons as this book explains and do things to boost your immune system like taking Astragalus. Avoiding aluminum based anti-deodorants will help too, by keeping your lymph system healthy. Once that aluminum soaks into your underarms, it poisons your lymph glands and nodes. Your lymph system is part of your immune system.

If you just have to use drugs, ask your doctor to prescribe you Colchicine. It is taken when you feel a gout attack coming on. Otherwise, you'll be taking gout medication every day to prevent gout until you get yourself completely cured.

Another thing you can do to cure yourself of Gout, even if you've done everything you know to do so far, is to drink high alkaline water. To create high alkaline water, it's best to use filtered water from a fluoride filter or osmosis water filtration system, then add some pH drops to that filtered water. The filters take out all that acidic chlorine and fluoride and other toxins. That removes the bitter taste of tap water and your water's pH becomes 7.0 or so; which is alkaline. Then if you add pH drops to that filtered water, the pH rises to 7.5 – 8.0 or so. Drinking 1-ounce of high alkaline water per 2 pounds of body weight daily will soon reverse the acidic state that you slowly put your body in over the years. It is more economical to just drink ½ teaspoon baking soda with 4-6 ounces of water 2-5x a day to cure your gout and all diseases.

This ripe for disease acidic state is created by regular consumption of animal products and sugars. Face the facts. Gout is the effect of overproduction of Uric ACID crystals. Did you get that? Uric ACID! And of course, those crystals rely on that acidic state to survive and multiply. That high alkaline water goes right through your kidneys! And as it does, it reverses the acidic state of your kidneys. And as your kidneys slowly create the contents of your blood, that blood is a more alkaline blood. And that blood begins to flow throughout your entire body; alkalizing your entire body over time.

Depending on how many animal products and sugar you continue to consume, you should reverse the acidic state of your body in 3 or 4 months on average. And the gout fades away and becomes just a memory!

Another problem kidney patients usually face is heart disease.

Heart disease – Basically, you need to take Magnesium, Fish oil and Flax seed oil. Your heart needs calcium to contract and Magnesium to relax your heart. This produces normal heart rhythms. Take 250-400mg daily for a few weeks. Then go to a maintenance dose of 250mg every other day.

Co-Q10 helps make your veins and arteries more elastic, which helps cure hardening of the arteries. Fish oil produces the same effect by emulsifying the fats and plaque that build up in your arteries and promote atherosclerosis. Take 100-150mg Co-Q10 daily and at least 1000mg fish or Flax seed oil daily. Fish oil and Flax seed oil help your heart and blood pressure because they contain Omega-3 fatty acid. Fish oil helps improve circulation. Omega-3 also reduces sudden death from cardiac arrhythmias. Fish oil also reduces triglycerides levels and helps stabilize blood clotting mechanisms; which prevents blood clots, a major cause of heart attacks and strokes. Fish oil "thins" the blood.

Niacin helps clean out your veins and arteries of plaque and other debris in your blood. Taking Fish oil and niacin can cure heart disease caused by plaque and hardening of the arteries. You need to take large doses of niacin to do this, but you run into a peculiar problem known as the red flush. Red flush is caused by doses of niacin as low as 25mg. This red flush is caused by the niacin expanding your capillaries to twice their normal size; allowing more blood flow to the surface of the skin. Be glad when you get it! This is the proof of the niacin working. By expanding your capillaries, your blood is able to carry a lot of toxins out of your body. To increase your dose of niacin, do this:

Start with 25mg niacin 2-3 times a day. When you no longer get the red flush, increase the dose to 50mg 2-3 times a day. Repeat this until you are at 100mg 2-3 times a day. Then up the dose by 50mg each time until you no longer get the red flush. You can do this all the way up to 500mg.

Just remember that if you stop taking niacin for a while, don't start back taking the same dose as you were. The red flush could very well be painful instead of warming and slightly uncomfortable.

When I was first diagnosed with chronic kidney disease, my EKG showed that I had an enlarged heart. I had trouble breathing more than a few times in those months just prior to and after that EKG. Doctors only expected it to get worse, not better. Because of the way I have eaten the past 30 years, I don't have a problem with cholesterol. But I cured myself of an enlarged heart by doing the same things I told you here about getting rid of the poisons I was consuming. I asked Dr. Allen if I could get another EKG to see if I had damaged my heart by having long term high blood pressure. My EKG was very good. I had an EKG again in 2011 and it was almost perfect.

Be sure to do things for **Stress** to help minimize putting harmful pressure on your heart and circulatory system. And of course, exercise regularly, drink lots of pure water and eat as many fresh fruits and vegetables as you can. And, since people often mistake heartburn (acid reflux) as a heart attack, be sure to use Apple Cider Vinegar and baking soda to cure your Acid Reflux heartburn.

Cardiovascular disease is the leading cause of death in the USA, even though most heart disease is preventable. Use this book to help you do so.

And do I have to tell you to stop smoking or stop drinking alcohol? These are the only 2 poisons that doctors will warn you about. If you gotta drink, don't drink in excess. That means, no more than 2-ounces in a 24 hour period, no more than 3 or 4 times a week. Alcohol is acidic and cigarettes are packed with poisons. I just went ahead and mentioned this in case some of you might tell yourself it's OK to smoke cigarettes and drink alcohol if I didn't mention it.

So that's about it for the information you need to avoid dialysis and most likely cure yourself of kidney disease and the diseases that develop as a result of the progression of your chronic kidney disease.

I didn't want to sound preachy or that I was on a pedestal talking down to you. I just wanted to share with as many people as I could, about the incredible journey I went on once my kidneys blew out in late 2006.

I never set out to cure myself of arthritis, gout, headaches or anything. I only wanted to try and help my kidneys get better to avoid going on dialysis and dying. I cured myself of every disease I had. So what I did cured every disease and medical condition I had, except for high blood pressure.

The damage to my kidneys caused my kidneys to stop releasing hormones that help control blood pressure. Everything is fixed and I have eliminated at least 90% of the poisons that I didn't even call poisons until the end of 2006 going into 2007. So I put all the information I needed to cure myself of all those diseases and medical conditions in this book. And **90% of this book came from my memory in my head, because I know all this stuff so well now.**

It is real frustrating to have such great and powerful knowledge and have it almost completely ignored. But no one is picking on just me! The one doctor who I found is keeping people off dialysis, is being ignored too; Dr. David Moskowitz. He is talked about in depth in Self-Care Health Care Guide and also in How to Avoid Dialysis and Cure Kidney Disease.

Dr. Moskowitz turned over the data for his proven treatments to arrest kidney disease, to the National Institute of Health. It is their job to get this information to this nation's medical profession to put into practice. But even though Dr. Moskowitz's treatment would have saved the government $500 Billion in just the past 10 years alone, to this day, the NIH claims they don't even know about Dr. Moskowitz's treatments and don't even know what they are.

And before that, the VA hospital Dr. Moskowitz worked at and had kept over 1000 US War Veterans off dialysis for up to 11 years, put an end to Dr. Moskowitz's treatments. And one by one they all got worse and worse, to the point that Dr. Moskowitz could not bear to continue watching it. So he resigned from that VA hospital. And when my doctors began to realize that I was curing myself, they sent me certified letters stating that they would no longer be my doctors. They were quite nasty about it when I called them to ask what was really going on with all that.

So in this next chapter I am going to give you the details of what I went through after doctors said I would be dead or on dialysis by 2008 or 2009.

The only chance beyond that was to be one of the rare few that receive a kidney transplant. But even that will only give you 10 years or so. Some even die from the transplant soon after it is done. And since no one ever dealt with the CAUSE of their kidney disease, that wreck-less consumption of poisons for pleasure and sensation and not for nutrition will also disease your new kidney.

I can never get off this powerful principle. Deal with the CAUSE.

Deal with the CAUSE. Deal with the CAUSE.

Doctors TREAT your diseases. But the ONLY way I will TREAT your diseases is to help you get rid of all disease and live free of disease from now on.

Let old age be your CAUSE of death, not disease.

Because there IS a cure for ALL disease. And in this next chapter, I am going to tell you how I discovered the cure for all disease, except for some of the 20% caused by germs and viruses.

Actually, I am going to tell you how I was FORCED to discover the cure for all disease or die. It is just as shocking and overwhelming to me today as it was when I first realized what I had discovered and done.

12 - How I Discovered the Cure For All Disease

Well, here we are on chapter 12, the chapter I have referred to a few times in previous chapters. This is where I tell my story about how I came to know most of the facts and truths I have been writing in this book and sharing with people in my daily life. Now I know that most of you have been wondering about some things. Like, how did I come to know all these things I'm talking about in this book? What are my credentials? Why should you listen to me, much less believe me? Do I think I'm smarter than doctors? And...probably a few other questions like that.

You may have noticed that I didn't give you information about my education or college degrees, where I studied medicine and other things like that. The reason is because I am not a licensed doctor, have no medical degree or college degree. And I only think I'm smarter than doctors when it comes to curing disease. I've cured many chronic diseases. All doctors combined ZERO.

I AM smarter than all doctors when it comes to curing disease. I proved that first, then started admitting it. You will understand how true that is just by accepting the facts as they are. It's up to you to decide who to believe when it comes to the subject of cures for disease. You can keep listening to doctors who don't have any cures OR you might consider listening to someone whose knowledge has actually cured people of chronic diseases and medical conditions. Listen to those who have cured disease! I'm not really asking you to choose. Hey, if your doctor already cured you, you don't need my help. Let me know. I honestly don't know of anyone who has been cured by a doctor. And boy I have looked and looked. You do that when your life is on the line.

I'm a pretty open minded person. So I'll try something to see if it works as it says. I often joke that if clipping clothes pins to my nose will cure me of a disease, I'll wear clothes pins on my nose until I'm cured. Ha ha! An open mind is a requirement if you're going to prevent disease and cure yourself of disease. Now, if you have clothes pins on your nose, please, take them off!

The story leading up to this book really began in 1981 when I started taking an interest in eating a little healthier and began gardening organically. I learned a lot of wonderful things over the years since then. But I didn't have any proof there were any cures. I never got a cure for anything when I was growing up. I never heard of doctors curing anyone of anything either. But like most everyone in this country, when you get sick you go to the doctor. So when I made my first doctor's appointment in October 2006 I assumed I would be cured by the doctors. I couldn't wait to get to the doctor, as bad as I felt. I never had a need for them, except for one trip to the emergency room in 1996 for my 3rd bladder stone attack, a broken collar bone and knee surgery as a teenager.

I only had the flu for 4 days one time from 1981 up to this very day too. So my experience with sickness was limited to those events and a lifetime of occasional headaches and my 20 year ordeals with heartburn, arthritis, bleeding gums and intestines and dandruff. I developed heart disease, gout, near diabetes, erectile dysfunction and chronic kidney disease during 2005-2006.

From about 2000 until late 2006, I blindly poisoned myself with at least 3 sodas a day, sometimes adding an extra icy quart of soda pop to that total, a 20-ounce Gatorade every day, a quart of the most popular brand cranberry juice; along with my sugary quart of tea a day at meals. I didn't start out drinking all that every day back in 2000. I gradually built that entire mess of bad habits for a couple of years and then sometime in 2003 I was drinking all that soda, juice, Gatorade and sweet tea. Big deal huh?

Since I trusted those companies that produce those products, the only thing I thought was how brilliant I was for drinking all that cancer fighting tea, that healthy ole cranberry juice and good ole Gatorade to get my electrolytes. I never thought for a minute that any of those drinks were hurting me in any way. Healthy organic food and healthy drinks. Ah, is this Heaven! I really thought I was doing great. But in early 2006 I started feeling like crap. My lower back would ache all the time and I got to feeling more and more lethargic, run down.

I had some back problems before 2006, but always managed to work them out within a few days. This never-ending back pain was confusing me, since it was not going away. I continued to do what I could for back pain. I tried everything I could think of to relieve the pain in my lower back. I used an inversion table, Gazelle, lifting weights, walking, heating pad, massages and lots more. But that aching back pain continued to persist.

Now when June came that year, 2006, my throat began to bleed one afternoon. I felt something tickle my throat, and when I coughed I hacked out blood. I thought it was my gums bleeding as they use to do every day. But when I started to try and isolate where the blood was coming from, I realized it was coming from my throat. I got a bit scared when I realized that I must have throat cancer. I kept trying to clear the blood out of my mouth and throat, but it kept coming. My throat bled and bled for 16 straight hours. I laid on the bed with a large plastic blue glass and spit blood in it for that entire 16 hours. I spit out a lot of clots, coagulated blood, in that 16 hours. I fell asleep finally and when I woke up, my throat wasn't bleeding. I drank water to wash the blood taste out of my mouth and that was the end of it for the time being.

After that throat bleeding episode in June, I still had the pain in my lower back. It would get worse, then better, then worse again until the first week of October 2006. I woke up one night right after 2 A.M. to go to the bathroom. I had to piss so bad I was hurting to go. As I was pissing, I felt like I was going to pass out and as I did, I looked down and saw my pee was real pink to reddish in the toilet and all the sudden a clump comes out and drops in the toilet. I dropped to my knees instantly, fell on my face and started to pass out. I regained my vision before I completely blacked out and started crawling out of the bathroom, through our band room, to my bed. I started mumbling to my wife, who was asleep, "Sandra, Sandra. Help me. Help me".

She woke up and freaked out at what she saw, but tried to help me. She helped me up and helped me lay down on the bed. I had no idea what was wrong with me, what caused it or what to do for myself. So I just laid in bed while my wife sat up the rest of the night to keep an eye on me in case anything else happened, worse than what had already occurred. I fell asleep a couple of hours later and my wife dosed off once she saw me fall asleep. Neither one of us slept very long.

We got up for the day between 6 and 7 A.M. And that's when the evil fun really got going. I spent the next week standing over the toilet at first. Then I had to start sitting on the toilet to try and pee dozens of times a day, since I was getting tired of standing half the day trying to pee. I didn't really need to pee all the time. It just felt like I needed to. You know how it is. You take a leak to relieve yourself. But no matter how much I tried to relieve myself, relief never came that week. I barely slept. On my best days that week I would sleep maybe 2-3 hours. I would try to go to sleep. But I would just lay in bed unable to fall asleep and end up getting up and standing over the toilet waiting for some relief. But no relief.

I can't pinpoint whether it was just a week or more than a week this went on while I waited for the day of my first doctor's appointment in about 30 years. I was dazed and shocked and in my own little world, just hoping for a few seconds of relief from the constant body aches and impulses to pee dozens of times a day. My wife was in shock too. She had never seen me in that shape and was just so naive about how bad a shape I was in. And she had been with me the whole time I had my four bladder stone attacks 10 years earlier from 1993-1996. We were both scared because we didn't know what was going on.

I tried to get some sleep in my own bed, then another bed. I tried falling asleep on the couch, the floor and other places, but I couldn't sleep. I began peeing in a cup so I could see if my pee had blood in it and to catch any blood clots if I peed out any more. I had blood in my pee a few times that first week or two, but only peed blood clots that first night, then once more. I was doing everything I could think of to help myself, but nothing was really helping. It was tough to find anything to eat, because I had pretty much lost my appetite. About the only thing I could stand to eat was canned whole kernel corn.

So I ate corn every day and sipped a little tea until I couldn't stand to eat any more. Believe me, it wasn't much food. I never ate a whole can at one time. The best I ever felt for a moment or two here and there was when I would do some sit ups with the new AB Chair I received the day after I pissed those first blood clots. I would do 2-3 hundred a day. Anything to lessen the discomfort and pain for even a moment here and there! Using that AB Chair was the only real relief I got until I drank some lemon balm tea.

After about a week or more had passed with me doing the same daily routine of trying to pee, trying to sleep and trying all kinds of things to feel better...I asked my wife if there was anything she could think of that we had NOT tried. While she was thinking about that I said "What about lemon balm tea?" Then I said "No, I don't see how that would help. But hey, let's try some anyway."

Besides the lower back pain and other body aches, I even felt pain and discomfort from my crotch all the way to my throat the whole time. I had gotten use to all of it by the time I tried the lemon balm tea. My stomach ached the whole time too. My wife made me the cup of lemon balm tea and when I took the first drink, I could feel that lemon balm tea going down my throat, down my chest, hitting my stomach and beyond. Boy did that feel good.

At first I just thought that I was feeling the heat from the tea. But I actually started to feel better. I could hardly believe it! Then I got to thinking.... Maybe I just think I'm feeling better? Maybe I just want to think the lemon balm tea helped? But since it made me feel the best I had felt in almost two weeks, I drank two more cups that day and felt better after each cup. As I kept pissing into a clear glass cup, I noticed there wasn't blood in my pee. My pee wasn't pinkish like it had been the whole time those two weeks.

So I kept drinking cups of lemon balm tea; at least 4 or 5 cups a day. I could hardly resist drinking it because I was so beat down, sick, hurting, aching, dazed, scared and as tired as I have ever been. I even began to think I was going to be OK and even thought about canceling the doctor's appointment. But since I was far from being well, I kept that doctor's appointment.

Now before I go on, let me tell you what my wife began to notice about my body. She noticed that I had about a dozen bruises on my back. As we both began to look for more bruises we found the most obvious bruise which was on my right side just below my ribs, bruises on my arms here and there and other places. There was about 15-20 bruises total. I wondered what the heck was going on with all those bruises. I hadn't done anything to get all those bruises!

So where'd they come from? What caused them? It was a few weeks before I finally realized what had caused them. My doctor's appointment is the next thing that happened. So, I'll tell you what caused those bruises when I get to the time I found out a few weeks later.

When I got to the doctor's office, which is a local well-known medical clinic a block from the hospital, the doctor didn't really know what was wrong with me exactly. So he did some tests. He did tell me that day that I had high blood pressure and he would give me something for that high blood pressure. As I was leaving, the doctor gave me some samples of the medication he thought I should take. When he handed me the medication I asked him "How long do I need to take this?" The doctor replied "The rest of your life." I was dumb founded immediately. Here I had been free of serious sickness for decades and the doctor was telling me I would have to take drugs for the rest of my life! Holy crap, I thought! I also thought that maybe when he gets my test results back he'll change his tune. I couldn't imagine being on drugs the rest of my life.

Everyone had made such a big deal about me being on drugs from age 19-26 that it was weird hearing anyone tell me I NEEDED to take drugs the rest of my life. I felt like I should have just stayed on drugs in the first place and never got off them. I couldn't handle the thought of doing drugs. So it took me a couple of days to actually start taking the drugs he had given me.

I was taking Nisoldipine. It made me feel yucky. But I kept taking it anyway, since that's all I had. The doctor's office called the day after my appointment and told me that it looks like I have kidney disease and that I needed to come back in within the next two weeks. So as I waited to go back to the doctor, I took my Nisoldipine and continued drinking lemon balm tea and using my new AB Chair; working on trying to feel better.

My test results revealed that my creatinine was 2.9 and so was my Potassium. Normal creatinine for a male is 1.5. Normal Potassium level is between 3.6 and 5.2. So my creatinine proved I had kidney disease for at least 14 months prior to these tests; which would be about August 2005. My identical 2.9 Potassium level was well below normal, so the doctor gave me a prescription for high potency Potassium. This went a long ways in relieving the immense tension I had been feeling for the past 3 weeks. I went from being iron man to Gumby the rubber man. Once I had taken all of that prescription I felt better but still had a lot of nervous tension. It wasn't something I had felt before my whole life. It turned out to be my blood pressure going as high as 240/140 a lot. While all this was going on with me I also had to deal with my mother being in the hospital in Intensive Care, on her death bed.

I went to my second doctor's appointment about the 25th of October and the doctor said he was scheduling 2 CAT scans for me to find out if I had kidney stones or anything else wrong in my lower torso. I told him that there was no way I could have kidney stones because I take Magnesium regularly. But he insisted. So I went along. But when I went to the office that handled the scheduling for the CAT scans, I told them I would have to know how much it was going to cost before I could agree to them. I told them if they cost too much then I'll just have to do without them if I couldn't afford them.

They had never had anyone ask them this. The lady called several people in the clinic. Then called the hospital that actually did the CAT scans, but no one could tell me the cost of the CAT scans. I told them I would have to know before I could agree to take the CAT scans. They said they would have to call me and let me know when they found out. I thought that was ridiculous!

They called the next day and said it would be $1100. So I refused and said I guess I'll just have to die since I can't afford it. My next doctor's appointment was a few days before Christmas. But in the meantime, some very bad things happened and I was about to start what turned out to be what saved my life.

My mother had been in a nursing home for 20 months when she had to be rushed to the hospital and put on a ventilator to stay alive. Her heart had given out; mostly because she was 85 years old. This was almost a month later to the day after my kidneys failed around October 6, 2006. I was pretty sure this was the end for my mother, so my wife and I went to the hospital every day to stay with her as long as they would let us. One of those first days I was standing at the end of my mother's bed and my wife asked "Why are your lips so dark red?" I immediately wiped my finger across my lips and said "Oh no! That's blood." And sure enough my throat starting bleeding again like it did back in early summer for 16-18 straight hours. I got scared about this.

Cold and flu season was in full swing and the thought of me catching a cold was terrifying. Just a tiny cough had started both throat bleeding episodes. I made my wife go straight to the shower as soon as she walked in the door from work, to try and wash off any cold or flu germs she might have on her clothes or body; since her work brings her in direct contact with many people every day.

Now while my mother was in the hospital for those last 10 days of her life, I was talking to the head nurse there named Pat. My Aunt Lora May Talley had been her usual hateful self and had taken control over who could see my mother or get any information on her condition. So I was trying to find out how such a bizarre thing could happen. Pat was helping me get that situation corrected. They ended up putting me as the person to represent my own mother and I put a password to keep Lora May from causing any more trouble.

I was use to her hatefulness. But I just wasn't in the mood for it for obvious reasons. Lora May had given me a scolding speech a few days earlier about how the only thing to do was pull the plug on my mother and let her die. I was never going to do that. My only thoughts were to fight for her life. I am always in favor of Life. As Pat and I were talking about all this, I mentioned that I had just been diagnosed with chronic kidney disease.

We got to talking about this and she told me her husband also had kidney disease. So I asked her what he was doing about it and did she know anything that could possibly help me. **Now what she was about to tell me didn't seem like it was all that important at the time, but it's what she told me that led me to the information that I know saved my life by arresting and reversing my chronic kidney disease.** She told me that what her husband was doing was taking ginger packs and putting them on his back where his kidneys are. **She said the ginger packs, poultice, draws the poisons out of his kidneys.**

This is what led me to saving my own life. Did ginger packs save my life? No. I never got that far. But as soon as Pat told me this I was extremely excited.

This was the first thing I had heard that would help someone with chronic kidney disease. The doctors only gave me dialysis and death within 2-3 years. As I began looking for the ginger root to do exactly what Pat had told me about, **I asked myself the question that is the question that actually ended up saving my life - What if you never put the poisons IN your body? Then you wouldn't have to get them out! So that's what I began to do and do so obsessively.** After all, 2-3 years to live doesn't give you any time to wait around for a cure or help. The only reason I valued what Pat told me was that it was the ONLY help I had gotten. So it was dialysis, death or ginger packs!

At the same time my mother passed away November 14 and that hit me hard. The day of her funeral it was around freezing with sleet and rain. So I couldn't even go to her funeral, since I couldn't risk exposing myself to weather that could give me a cold or the flu. Remember, my throat was bleeding and if I caught a cold, the coughing from that cold would keep my throat bleeding for days; enough to bleed to death. After my mom died, I dragged around in a daze, not caring much about how near death I was.

It was during those following days while I was wondering where the poisons came from that caused my kidneys to fail that I thought - I had eaten pretty healthy for decades, so this poisons idea wasn't making sense to me. It's right here where I realized some of the poisons I had overlooked were in those fruit juices I was drinking. I would get that wired up tense feeling after drinking juices. That's when I began to recognize that same feeling when I ate or drank other things. I didn't think they were poison at that time. I just didn't like that wired up tense feeling, no matter what was causing it. So I was getting serious about finding out what was causing that feeling.

I knew what I ate and drank to give me that feeling. But what was in those products that was THE cause of it? I began to form my own opinion, but didn't have any idea if I was right about the opinion I was forming. I was going to stick with my developing opinion until someone told me something better that would help me. As this opinion was just beginning, I went for my 3rd doctor's appointment and my 2nd blood tests to see how my kidneys were doing.

My test results came back December 26 and revealed that my creatinine was going up point 1 a month and was now 3.1. My Potassium was 5.7 after being 2.9 just 2 months ago. My BUN had gone up from 30 to 44 too. BUN is basic urea nitrogen, which basically is a sign of your kidney's inability to digest protein. As a result, my doctor insisted I should see Dr. Edwards, the clinic's nephrologist. That visit lasted over 2 hours. That's when they took my blood pressure and it was 240/140. I just sat there calmly and they were pretty frantic. The doctor said "Your blood pressure is dangerously high".

It was 240 over 140. So they started giving me Atenolol and had me put in under my tongue. The nurse would come back in about 20 minutes and take my blood pressure, leave the room, come back and give me some more Atenolol to put under my tongue. We went through this routine at least 3 times and finally they said I could leave. I was given a prescription and told to see Dr. Edwards as soon as possible. I still had that nervous tension that high blood pressure gives you. I didn't know it at the time, but that Atenolol they gave me doesn't really lower blood pressure. It only slows your heart down so your high blood pressure doesn't do as much damage to your organs. So you can see that yucky Nisoldipine let my blood pressure rise to 240/140 or more. All the Atenolol was doing was slowing my heart down.

During that visit, Dr. Forte did something that shocked me. He had always been a quiet man and said very little to me for the most part. I had made it a point not to tell him about the lemon balm tea stopping my internal bleeding and giving me such significant relief over the past 3 months. But I ended up saying something about it and he raised his voice in a snap and yelled angrily "Well, did your lemon balm tea tell you you have chronic kidney disease?" I stayed silent to keep him from blowing up even worse. I had kept my mouth shut about it all along because I was worried about making someone mad if I mentioned it. I never mentioned anything like that to him again.

I did what the doctor and nurses told me to do and that included taking the Nisoldipine and the 100mg Atenolol daily. The 100mg Atenolol was only suppose to slow my heart down to about 60 beats a minute, but ended up slowing my heart to 40 BPM. So they had to lower that to 50mg Atenolol. I told them I was gonna stop taking the Nisoldipine, since it was yucky and costs quite a bit. It was gonna cost over $1000 a year. I was paying cash for everything. So that cost was unreasonable to me and my cash. I worked with a nurse and we finally found a calcium channel blocker called Amlodipine for me to take, along with the 50mg Atenolol. But as December turned into January and into spring, I was busy doing everything I could do to help myself.

A lot of what I was doing was researching on the INTERNET, trying to find anything that might help me and what those things were and did for you. This was kind of hard because my eyes had gotten bad all the sudden because of my kidney failure and high blood pressure. I had to find my mother's reading glasses and use them to read anything on the INTERNET or food labels. I had no idea what, if anything, was going to help me; since doctors only gave me dialysis, death, drugs, tests and high doctor bills. So I worked hard on finding poisons in my food, drinks, hygiene items and water.

I admit, I became obsessed. But all my life I've been the best at most things I do; football, baseball, track, fastest runner, playing guitar, playing in bands and more. So I was gonna do the same about trying to save my own life and get rid of the poisons entering my body through my water, food, drinks and hygiene items. So as I waited for my appointment with Dr. Edwards, the clinic's nephrologist, I worked feverishly on this. Once I stopped drinking all the high fructose corn syrup soaked sodas and juices, I started feeling a lot better during those early months of 2007.

Besides starting my own personal war to eliminate high fructose corn syrup from my diet, I was doing lots and lots of other things too. We got our shower filter, then our fluoride water filter, stopped buying red meat, quit buying sugar, quit cooking with the microwave, changed to organic soaps, less toxic toothpaste and more; just in those first few months of all this. I realized it could all turn out to be a waste of time and money. But my money was no good to me dead. So I stuck with this obsession for the next few years.

Another obsession I quickly developed was taking my blood pressure! They recommended that I take it every day. But old obsession boy ME did it excessively. I took my blood pressure 30-40 times a day. I wanted to see what effect all kinds of activities and foods had on my blood pressure. But my actual blood pressure was taken following all the guidelines required to accurately take blood pressure, when I did it. They never follow these guidelines in the doctor's office or hospitals. So their results are near meaningless. My real blood pressure stayed about 160-180 over 90-110 the first 3 months of 2007, taking 50mg Atenolol and 10mg Amlodipine daily.

I was also working on my high Potassium and had only my Potassium tested every couple of weeks until my appointment with Dr. Edwards. When I finally got to that appointment with Dr. Edwards, a nephrologist, I was scared about seeing how much worse my kidneys were than back in December. I expected my creatinine to be up from 3.1 to at least 3.5 and bring me less than 2 years from having to go on dialysis.

When the day of my appointment came it was the first week of April and I was glad I was going to get some real help now. Dr. Edwards ordered more blood tests, a urinalysis and prescribed me Clonidine to go along with the Amlodipine and Atenolol I was already taking. He also asked me to take my blood pressure every day and give him the results for the next two weeks once I had them. But in the meantime, my test results came back. I had some protein in my urine and my Potassium was still high at 5.5. Everything else was normal, except my BUN and creatinine; which are the two main factors doctors use to determine kidney function. My BUN had gone down from 44 in December to just 27 and my creatinine, instead of going up to 3.5 as the doctors said it would, went DOWN, all the way down to 2.6! That was a 9 month swing in my favor plus the last 4 months to boot! I couldn't believe it and really wasn't sure what had caused this human miracle or if it would last!

I reported my daily blood pressure readings to Dr. Edwards two weeks later as he had asked for. My overall average blood pressure was 145/75 for the two weeks, but my pulse was just 55. So they said to come back and see Dr. Edwards in a year. But in the meantime, I continued to see Dr. Forte and talk to one male nurse named Matt. I didn't like the idea of being tied to doctors, so I didn't go back for 6 months. I don't have records covering this one year from mid April 2007 until March 2008.

One bizarre thing did happen during this time. When I went back to see Dr. Forte, some female nurse was doing the usual line of questions and I was answering them as I always did. But then she asks "Do you believe you have chronic kidney disease?" I hesitated, and smiled, thinking... is this a real question or a trick question? Since the doctors said that I did, I thought it was settled. I answered her and said "That's what the doctors say." She then typed for a minute or so into her laptop. I later found out she had not recorded what I actually said. She put in my medical records that I did not believe I had chronic kidney disease and that I believed I could heal myself of my chronic kidney disease. I only found out because I allowed DHS to look at my medical records in an effort to get some help paying for the expensive drugs I had to take.

They wanted me to go see a psychiatrist. I was as puzzled as I could be. And even more so since it wasn't standard procedure. So I demanded a copy of my medical records from the clinic I was going to. I read through my medical records and that's how I found out about this.

Hey! Sure I'm crazy IF I think I can cure myself of a disease that I don't even believe I have, according to Nurse Fibber! LOL Problem was, I never even thought such a thing, much less SAID it. I realized she had asked the question because I had said I was going to be cured. But that was only because I had not accepted what they said about no one ever being cured or getting better with chronic kidney disease. It was also because I thought they were going to cure me. I didn't know doctors have no cures until then. All I cared about was being cured and being well. I didn't realize yet that I was never going to get any help for my kidneys at that clinic or from those doctors.

But the next time I went back to the doctor, after seeing that garbage on my medical records, I spoke to Nurse Fibber about what she wrote. She insisted that she only wrote what I said. Bah hum bug! When the only nurse that had helped me stepped in, he explained that they can't remove anything from my medical records, but they can put a note saying the patient never actually said that. So I dropped it.

During that year from April 2007 to March 2008, I kept doing the drugs for high blood pressure; since they said if I didn't, my kidneys would get worse even faster than they had so far. But I worked on getting rid of the poisons in my food, drinks and personal hygiene items. Remember, once I got the fluoride water filter and the shower filter in early 2007, my water was pure and safe; except for about 10% of the chlorine and all the fluoride in the shower water.

So I worked on avoiding the poisons in our food, drinks and hygiene items and drank at least 3 quarts of water a day. I also drank Goji, Mangosteen and Noni juice a lot. I ate lots of fruits and vegetables, fish, chicken and turkey, but no red meat or pork to speak of. I was getting depressed from time to time because the doctors had done nothing for my kidneys; only for the high blood pressure that caused the chronic kidney disease.

You gotta remember that my mother had been in a nursing home for the past 21 months, then died the month after I was diagnosed with chronic kidney disease. My mother had to file for bankruptcy because Regions Bank would not take payments from me when my mother became unable to care for herself at all; as though this kinda thing was unheard of to Regions Bank. We barely saved the house from auction 9 months before my mom passed. All the doctors said I would be dead or on dialysis by 2008 and no later than 2009.

There was no hope for any future for me and I was all on my own to save my own life without any real help from anybody. You talk about pressure! I just want you to know what I went through while I was saving my own life, without knowing that I was. Who was I to say doctors were wrong? I was a dying man with just a couple of years left to live. I kept on taking my blood pressure a few dozen times a day until my next visit to Dr. Edwards in March 2008.

I had gotten to where when I went to the doctor I would ask "Is this the visit where you finally help me with my kidneys?" But that day never came. When I went to see Dr. Edwards the second time it was kinda awkward. I asked him about doing herbal cleanses and taking herbs. He said he had never studied herbs. Now if you know herbs are medicine, which they are, then you know Dr. Edwards told me that he had never studied medicine; which is actually true.

Dr. Edwards ordered more tests to test my kidney function again and to test me for PTH, parathyroid hormone levels. The tests came back showing my PTH levels were high. But my CMP, complete metabolic panel, results on March 31, 2008 shocked me. My creatinine had gone down from 2.6 in April 2007 to 2.2.

Remember, my creatinine was 3.1 on December 26, 2006. So instead of my creatinine being 4.6 in March 2008 as doctors insisted it would be, my creatinine was down to 2.2. I had added 24 months to my life already. Wow! How did that happen? My Potassium was also down to 4.1 compared to 5.5 a year earlier and marked the first time my Potassium had been in the normal range since my kidneys failed over 18 months earlier.

When the nurse called me to give me the results, she said I needed to take some new drug called something like Calcitril. She said Dr. Edwards was prescribing it to bring down my PTH levels. I said OK, but wanted to make sure there wasn't anything natural to help before I agree to any more drugs. I called the nurse back a few days later and discussed the possibility of taking calcium supplements instead of the drug. She was against that, but said she would ask

Dr. Edwards and get back to me.

See, your PTH levels rise if your body's parathyroid glands detect low calcium levels in your blood. Problem was, that my calcium was always mid-range normal. And also, the Amlodipine I was taking was a calcium channel blocker. It was blocking calcium from getting into my heart to keep my heart from retracting as hard, thus lowering my blood pressure. In other words, the Amlodipine was the cause of the high PTH levels. So I decided to find a way to stop taking the Amlodipine to solve this problem by eliminating the cause.

Now, since most of you probably don't know, a person with chronic kidney disease gets worse progressively. Your creatinine increases and your skin itches more and more because of it. You lose your appetite. You become anemic. Your ankles, face and other places get swollen because your kidneys aren't removing fluids from your body properly. And your metabolics get more and more out of whack until this and the skin itching can only be relieved by dialysis. You also grow closer and closer to becoming a diabetic and almost always do. So I had to work on preventing diabetes too.

When I called the clinic to find out why I hadn't heard from the nurse about that PTH thing, they wouldn't talk to me and made excuses. I was trying also to see when Dr. Edwards wanted me to come back to see him. But the end of May I received 2 certified letters from both of my doctors at that clinic. They both said that within 30 days they would no longer be my doctors and that they would forward my medical records to the doctor of my choice. Dr. Edwards stated that this action was "due to non-compliance and general resistance to his recommendations for your care."

That pissed me off and shocked me at first. It was ridiculous though because I had done everything they told me to do except for jumping right on that last drug Dr. Edwards had wanted me to take. Asking questions isn't resistance. Seeking alternatives isn't either. So it became clear to me that it had to be over me getting better by doing things for myself, while they demonstrated their helpless and unwilling interest in my health; much less helping me get better.

I called them and tried to talk to them and they were mean, hateful and belligerent. I was calling to ask when I could come and pick up 2 of my prescriptions that came straight from the manufacturer to the doctor's office and to get my other prescriptions to be refilled. But they refused and told me not to call again or they would have me arrested. So I dropped it and never talked to them again. I did talk to a wonderful person I had become friends with in the business office, Carolyn. She let me talk to her about paying Clopton Clinic the money I still owed them; which I paid in full with cash. So for all of June, July and 12 days of August I had no doctor or prescriptions and was all by myself again, still trying to save my own life without any help from doctors.

I heard there was a free church clinic in the old Holiday Inn building down town. So I gave them a call and learned I qualified to come there. My appointment was for August 12, 2008. When I got there for my appointment I was surprised to see that a girl friend, not girlfriend, was working there. So I talked with her about when we were in high school, who she married and if she had any kids and about my visit there. Everybody was real nice to me. My visit went real well. It was pretty uneventful. But at least I had a doctor again, after being thrown out of Clopton Clinic for getting better.

I did have my blood tested and the results came back a couple of days later. My Potassium was just 4.3. My BUN had dropped to 24 and my creatinine was 2.37; which was slightly above my last result of 2.1 five months earlier. I was relieved to find this out. I scheduled my next appointment for September. But a few days after my first appointment I made a surprise discovery.

I had been searching the INTERNET for almost two years for a cure for my chronic kidney disease, but hadn't found one. Actually, I hadn't even come close to finding a cure. I hadn't even found anyone claiming to cure kidney disease. All I had found so far was a book by a great pioneering doctor from John Hopkins Medical Center who had done clinical trials limiting his patients to 20 grams of protein daily to slow down the progression of kidney disease. His name was Mackenzie Walser. I found his book titled "Coping With Kidney Disease – A 12-Step Treatment Program to Help You Avoid Dialysis" and I ordered it from Amazon.com. What Dr. Walser had done is develop a program based on a British program that was a no protein diet. Dr. Walser's program was based on a 20 grams of protein daily diet.

I read the book and started to follow his program. I had trouble sticking with the 20 grams of protein daily. But I worked on limiting my protein, but could never get by with just 20 grams of protein daily. I had been working on this for over a year by the time I had my first appointment at the church health clinic. My tests results proved Dr. Walser's program was helping me because my BUN was down to 24.

After my first appointment on August 12, 2008, I was searching the INTERNET for the part of the title of Dr. Walser's book "avoiding dialysis". Much to my surprise, there was a new search result besides Dr. Walser's book. It was for GenoMed. I read over the site and saw they claimed to have superior clinical outcomes for several chronic conditions which included kidney disease caused by hypertension. I figured I could debunk that garbage quickly. So while I was reading over the web site, I found an email address I could contact them at about participating in their superior clinical outcome program.

I knew I was gonna get some dumb reply about worshiping the doctor while I paid him huge amounts of money in my quest to save my life. I had emailed the top dog at GenoMed, Dr. David Moskowitz on August 21; just 9 days after my first appointment at the church clinic. Dr. Moskowitz said he could help me but that we needed to act quickly since my creatinine was currently 2.37.

By the fourth email, Dr. Moskowitz had laid out what I needed and told me to give the information to my doctor at the church clinic, Dr. Pyle. I didn't really understand the program at this time, but took the information with me at my next appointment at the church clinic. But before I got to my appointment, I received notice that I had been approved for Medicaid. I had applied almost 18 months ago to get some help paying my $300+ monthly drug bill. DHS told me repeatedly that the only way I could get that kind of help was to apply for Medicaid. They wanted me to apply for Food Stamps, but that was ridiculous.

I only needed some help with that high monthly drug bill! As a result of me receiving approval for Medicaid, I no longer qualified for the church health clinic. So when I went for my second and last appointment there, I told them I couldn't come back any more.

While I was there, Dr. Pyle and I talked about what I needed for his program, but Dr. Pyle explained how he couldn't start me on the drugs Dr. Moskowitz ordered, since Dr. Pyle could not be my doctor any more. But Dr. Pyle did try to get me in to see a doctor who was a friend of his, Dr. Henry Allen. As we were talking, Dr. Pyle happened to mention how he and his friends use to come out to the fairgrounds and watch us play baseball. I said "Really? Who were you going out there to watch?" Dr. Pyle said "You. You were the best player. We went out there to see you." I was pleasantly surprised and told him "Gee thanks Dr. Pyle. Glad you enjoyed watching me play." I was surprised because all I had heard from the doctors was one asshole thing after another without any real sign of any doctor caring one damned bit!

Dr. Pyle said all he could do is give me a prescription for one drug Dr. Moskowitz suggested, since he wouldn't need to monitor me for that drug. I thanked Dr. Pyle and told him and his staff that I was sad that I couldn't come back and that I wished the greatest success for the wonderful service they were providing. So there I was, back to square one with no doctor. But with Medicaid approved for me then, I felt pretty good about finding a new doctor.

I contacted Dr. Allen's office which was White River Rural Health Clinic at that time. After talking to several employees there, they got all confused about what I had discussed with Dr. Pyle about what Dr. Moskowitz ordered for me. So they said they couldn't help me. I had DHS send me a complete list of doctors in my area who accepted Medicaid. I went through the whole list. I contacted 45 doctors and was turned down by each and every one of them.

They didn't want ANYTHING to do with someone getting cured and it didn't matter how offensive that was coming from all those doctors and staffs. It made it even more offensive after being kicked out of Clopton Clinic for getting better! I kept in contact with Dr. Moskowitz during September, October and November, always explaining how no doctor would go along with any plan to cure people or help them get better.

But toward the end of November I decided to call Dr. Pyle back. Dr. Pyle's real job is as Vice President of our main hospital. He volunteered at the church health clinic to work for free. So I contacted him at the hospital.

Dr. Pyle was kind to me. He said "Well, let me give them a call and see what I can do." I thought... Dr. Pyle had already done that and it didn't work out. So it's not gonna work this time either. But much to my surprise, White River Rural Health Clinic called me and asked for some personal information and made me an appointment as Dr. Pyle had asked them to do.

The appointment was for December 4. I contacted Dr. Moskowitz and told him the good news and he instructed me as to what I needed to tell the doctor. My visit with Dr. Allen went well and he prescribed the medications Dr. Moskowitz had ordered for me. I began taking them on December 8. Gee! So my six month ordeal since being thrown out of Clopton Clinic for getting better seemed to be over.

I figured I would get thrown out of White River Rural Health Clinic too. I hadn't had too much respect for doctors since becoming an adult and the bizarre backwards treatment and attitudes of Dr. Edwards and Forte had only made that worse and darker. But I kept thinking about friends of mine who are doctors and kept some positive hope because of them. I couldn't even imagine my friends, who became doctors, not caring about people.

So don't think I am prejudice against doctors just because the facts about them are negative most of the time. I had reserved myself to going along with doctors and keeping my mouth shut about natural things to them. After all, as much cash as I had to pay for whatever doctors did, I wasn't about to reject them to their faces or impede them from giving me the information or aid I paid for. I was just a helpless dying man who doctors only forecast for my future was death, dialysis or kidney transplant. All I cared about was saving my own life.

There had been no light at the end of the tunnel for me among doctors and the medical profession. That was about to all change. Two doctors joined my team, the Life team, the results matter team, the CURES are acceptable team, the Your Health now matters team...and maybe the Liars Can Now Eat Their Own poopie team! Ha ha!

I was now starting Dr. Moskowitz's program. This was a doctor who had already proven his treatments work through his work in clinical trials. I didn't have to listen to so many people tell me how crazy I am about using this doctor's treatment; like so many people have done about my gospel of poisons saturating our entire food, drinks and water supplies. Also, I had to sign a non-disclosure agreement agreeing not to talk about the specifics of his patented treatments and clinical trials.

But Dr. Moskowitz has given me specific permission as to what I CAN tell you. So I must stick to that agreement and those of you reading this will have to excuse me for being vague about this for this reason. Please.

After I had started the treatment on December 8, I went back to Dr. Allen's office to get my blood tested on the 15th. I had to do this while we were upping the dose of the medication as Dr. Moskowitz advised. Those tests showed my creatinine was 2.2 and my Potassium was 4.1. We were trying to see if the treatment was causing a rise in either one. Since all was good, we upped the dose. Next blood test was January 8. My creatinine was 2.13 and Potassium was 4.3. No problem. So we upped the dose again. Next test was January 30. My creatinine was 2.15 and my Potassium was 4.4. So no problem and we upped the dose again.

Next test was February 17. My creatinine was down to 2.0 and my Potassium was 4.6. So, like always, we upped the dose. Next test was March 9th. I was shocked to see that my creatinine was all the way down to 1.9! My Potassium was 4.6. So it was clear to me that this treatment was really working. But since the time I started this treatment on December 8, 2008 up until the second week of March 2009, I had been laying off the other drugs almost entirely. It was extremely difficult for me to get the drug I needed for this treatment. I had to get a new prescription almost every time we upped the dose and I had to find where to get it for a good price.

Paying $300+ a month just for this one drug was going to be a long term problem as far as I could see. Medicaid wouldn't pay a penny for that particular drug. It's not on their list. Yea I know, real dumb, right! But there was nothing I could do except keep on paying cash. Another problem during all these tests and upping the dose, was my blood pressure had gone up to 203/135! Yikes.

See, Dr. Moskowitz said there was chance, not a certainty, that I might be able to just end up on the one drug he was using to arrest my kidney disease. I was and still am against doing drugs. So I stay obsessed with doing as little drugs as I think I can get away with. What I do end up taking doesn't bother me though. I think about all those ibuprofen, aspirin, Aleve, Tylenol and antacids I do not take any more. So my drug intake is actually LESS than what it was the past 20 years.

With my blood pressure at 203/135, I didn't flip out or even get scared. I was just pissed because I knew I would have to get back to taking those other drugs along with the high doses of the drug at the center of my treatment. I didn't take my blood pressure again, because I knew my anger only made it go even higher. I did contact Dr. Moskowitz to see what he recommended. But it was only an improved version of what all I had been taking. None the less, we were both glad my creatinine was down to 1.9 and I had reached the dosage I needed to be on. What I already came to know was that, all you can do about high blood pressure is take more drugs if your blood pressure is high.

Doctors sure don't have a cure for high blood pressure. I'm working on that for myself, but think it was probably caused by gene mutation or DNA damage from high fructose corn syrup.

I went to work to find a way to get that one drug cheaper. I found a lot of places online that claimed they could help. I spent quite a bit of time reading all the terms and services available for discount drugs. The best one seemed to be RX OutReach. And it was in the same city Dr. Moskowitz was in and one of my favorite cities too. RX OutReach, www.rxoutreach.org, allows you to buy a 90 day supply of one medication for $20 and $55 for a 180 day supply. It doesn't matter the dosage or the frequency of the dose either. So even though my prescribed dosage for my main drug is 6x the normal dose, I still get it for those same prices.

I did have a problem at the very first because their pharmacy rejected my order because of the unusual high dosage. I gave a desperate plea to them to fill my order. They still refused. But I had my doctor send them a fax and got it all cleared up. So I got my order a few days after that. I tell ya. Something was always popping up as an obstacle to me trying to get well, no matter who, what, when or where I made the effort to get help from the medical profession!

Once I got all this tangled mess worked out about trying to get all the drugs I now needed, I felt I was in the best shape yet. I had to get back on the drugs I had backed off after starting the treatment. I had finally gotten a local doctor to help with all this. And, I had also solved a few other lesser problems.

But when I had my next blood test April 13, my creatinine had gone UP to 2.3 from 1.9 just five weeks earlier! I thought, oh my God, I've really messed up now! I was shattered. I thought the worst. After all, there had never been any real hope for me getting well. So I wasn't really surprised; just defeated in my quest to cure myself or at least never have to be on dialysis.

I figured that my blood pressure going up to 203/135 and probably being up for a few weeks, caused damage to my kidneys. So that was the explanation for my creatinine going up from 1.9 to 2.3 in just 5 weeks! That was 4x the rate of creatinine rising from kidney failure you are supposed to have. So I was scared as I waited for my next tests I insisted on just 3 weeks later. On May 4 my creatinine was holding at 2.3. BUN was 24 and Potassium was 4.5. This dumb founded me and neither Dr. Allen nor Dr. Moskowitz could explain what had or was happening. I had my theory, but couldn't be for sure.

But my next test about 2 months later, July 31, showed my creatinine was still holding at 2.3. There was no sign that my kidneys had actually gotten worse. I thought about this until sometime in the fall and finally concluded that my creatinine had gone down to 1.9, then back up to 2.3 in five weeks because I had gone back to taking Atenolol which slowed my heart down by about 1/3.

I concluded this as THE cause and realized that slowing my heart down made a point 3 difference and that there had been no further damage to my kidneys; much less, major damage. Then when I got my test results for December 10, I was convinced of this and breathed a big sigh of relief. I also breathed a gigantic sigh of relief because I was still alive at the end of 2009 and was not on dialysis either, as all the doctors insisted I would be! Now all I had to do was to maintain what I had achieved.

Back in June I had kinda fallen off the horse about avoiding high fructose corn syrup. I could barely say anything about it without people being totally disinterested and downright hateful a lot of times and crazy. So I gave up on that and started back not caring how much high fructose corn syrup I consumed. This went on for June, July and into August when I woke up with gout one morning in August 2009. I said oh no. I hope this goes away soon. It hurt so horrifyingly bad. So I stopped chugging down the high fructose corn syrup and ate extremely well again.

But that gout stayed with me for TWO WHOLE MONTHS. I yelled and screamed a lot and laid down most of the time. I was in such miserable pain that I couldn't even imagine how I could get to a doctor. Shoot, the 15 foot trip to the bathroom was filled with mind numbing pain, yelling and screaming and the horror of having to make that same trip back to the bed or lounger!

It was during this two month long affliction of gout that sealed the doom for high fructose corn syrup with me forever. And I mean FOREVER! I thought there might be another episode of gout even after I got off the high fructose corn syrup, to prove me wrong. But it never came. And I have not had any gout since. The doctor gave me some pills to take if I think gout is coming on; which I have used twice, but never did have gout. I took it as a precaution two times. I finally ended my gout by drinking baking soda water.

Another situation that was going on for most of this time was DHS fighting against me to keep me from getting what was lawfully and legally mine. Remember, I applied for Medicaid to get some help paying my $300+ monthly drug bill. Before I applied, I checked to see if I had a chance of qualifying. The terms state that if your disease is expected to last more than 12 months or end in death, then you qualify. And since doctors all claimed that all chronic kidney patients end up dead and their disease lasts more than 12 months, I knew I qualified. The word chronic clarifies that! But the phony government works AGAINST the People, not FOR the People. So I had to fight them for 18 months. Fortunately for me, I knew I qualified. So no matter what corrupt behavior DHS used, I knew to let it go and keep appealing.

Their goal is to force you to fight them on your death bed to get what is legally and lawfully yours! They hope to at least delay you from getting anything in hopes you will go ahead and die to avoid you getting what is legally and lawfully yours! This vile behavior should not be tolerated in America.

As 2009 ended and 2010 began, I decided I was going back to living my life after this 5 year ordeal of huge ups and downs with my life in the balance. I felt like I had kept my kidney disease in check and improved greatly. Just the fact that I went from 3.1 creatinine in December 2006 to 2.1 in December 2009 was incredible and unheard of in the medical profession anyway! My creatinine should have been 5.7 at that time, but was only 2.1! So I had already added SIX YEARS to my life. Three years I had not gotten worse, plus the three years it would take for me to need dialysis if I started getting worse after December 2009! And I had learned to control my Potassium.

And all that time I never developed any further symptoms of chronic kidney disease. I didn't get diabetes as they said I would either; although I did come very close to becoming a diabetic.

As a matter of fact, I had cured myself of headaches, heartburn, arthritis, dandruff, skin burns and itching and other things. But all I set out to do was save my own life by trying to cure myself of chronic kidney disease. I had all those other conditions and diseases for 20 years and I had never thought about dying from them. It was the chronic kidney disease that brought all the death and end of my life talk.

I had talked to our local newspaper and TV station about doing a story to save a lot of lives. But they claimed I hadn't done what I had done and that I couldn't claim I had since the medical profession didn't do it for me. It didn't even matter that three doctors could confirm it was true. They weren't reporting any cures! I thought how sick that really was. But I wasn't surprised at their rejection of reporting anything that would save lives or suffering. All they care about is reporting what big business does. They'll report the wonderful story of a child or adult that doctors "cured", but was back in remission and about to die and the new technology the medical profession buys to diagnose things better. But none of that will cure you.

I didn't try to talk them in to caring about people's lives. They made it more than clear that they would never even consider reporting anything that wasn't invented or done by the medical profession. **So, me being the only kidney patient in the area and being one of the rare rare ones in the entire country to arrest their kidney disease, was entirely meaningless and really offensive to them; our wonderful media!** Gag, hiccup, vomit!

I had proved the doctors wrong by living beyond 2009 and not going on dialysis. And I was determined to go ahead and go back to living my life without death hanging over my head and being my ONLY possible future according to the medical profession. I was still searching for a cure, but continuing Dr. Moskowitz's treatment program and following my own ways that reversed my kidney disease. I was still trying to figure out what I had done that helped, from anything that actually didn't help me at all. And I was still all alone on this. I mean, who COULD I talk to that could tell me how a chronic kidney patient

COULD get better or be cured?

I kept making regular searches on the INTERNET for this very thing; just as I had been doing since October 2006 when my kidneys failed. I thought I had found a cure when I ran across an advertisement on the INTERNET claiming an Australian man had cures, plural, for various kinds of chronic kidney disease. I was skeptical from the first. But at least he was saying what I wanted to hear... cures for kidney disease. So I forked out about $60 and bought his book and additional materials.

As I got to reading his book, I found many familiar things in his book. All of it was natural things and that was exactly what I believed in. I gathered the information to start his "cure" for my chronic kidney disease caused by hypertension. The cure instructed me to take vitamins and herbs that I was already taking, but in different doses. The main adjustment I had to make was taking 600mg of Alpha Lipoic Acid. So I ordered the Alpha Lipoic Acid in the 600mg size and begin to take it and the other items in his so-called cure.

I told my doctor, Dr. Allen, and he cautioned me not to take the 600mg Alpha Lipoic Acid. I told him I was going to go ahead and take it, since no one else had any ideas how to cure me. But I agreed to only take it for 3-4 months, even though the "cure" called for me to take 600mg Alpha Lipoic Acid until I was cured. I took my blood tests during that doctor's visit on February 10, 2010. My creatinine was down to 1.9 and my Potassium was 4.7. So I was ready to use this Australian man's "cure" to knock my kidney disease on out! I followed his "cure" until May 11.

When I went back to the doctor on May 11 I had my blood tested as I almost always did. My creatinine had gone UP to 2.2 and my Potassium was 5.5! Yikes! That was the first time my Potassium was out of the normal range in over three years. I was sure that I had messed up bad! But Dr. Allen told me that was exactly why he cautioned me about taking the 600mg Alpha Lipoic Acid. I knew Alpha Lipoic Acid caused your kidneys to reuse antioxidants, but never knew it did the same thing for Potassium and other vitamins and minerals. So there I was, back in trouble again without knowing what was going on. And it was pretty clear that this Australian guy's alleged "cure" was not a cure at all. I admit that it could help those who knew practically nothing, but didn't really add anything to what I was already doing.

As a matter of fact, this guy discredits himself by not cautioning you on the grave dangers that his "cures" cause. If your Potassium climbs to 6.0 or above, your heart will start to palpitate and it won't stop palpitating without emergency treatment. And there is nothing you can do to lower your Potassium in a few minutes, hours or even days. So his "cure" is quite dangerous and put my life in danger. Now I had to find a way to get my Potassium down and keep it from going any higher. I thought this guy's "cure" might have even damaged my kidneys. I was scared and on edge from time to time for the weeks following this blood test and wondered if I was going to get better or worse. So I scheduled more blood tests 6 weeks later on June 23.

My test results for June 23, 2010 revealed that my creatinine went up from 2.2 to 2.3. The HUGE surprise was that my Potassium had gone DOWN from 5.5 to 4.7! I was shocked. Dr. Allen was too, but not as much as I was. That's when he told me that was what he had cautioned me about the 600mg Alpha Lipoic Acid daily for. I thought that was really neat! But I told Dr. Allen right then and there that I had stopped taking the Alpha Lipoic Acid and that I was going to stop taking vitamins and herbs for at least a while.

After that, I felt I was at the end of my health improving and I was back on course heading back to dialysis and death; since my creatinine had gone up point 1 each and every month for the last four months. It went up from 1.9 in February to 2.3 in May. So I decided to give up and go ahead and live what little life I had left. I took another six month break from doctors and accepted that I was getting worse and dreaded ever going back to the doctor. I just didn't want to know that my kidneys were getting progressively worse. So I stayed away. I finally got the courage to go back to the doctor after Thanksgiving and made an appointment for December 21. I dreaded what my blood tests were going to be.

The next day the doctor's office called and said my creatinine was 1.8. I was so relieved, but only for a few seconds, when they told me my Potassium was 7.0! 7.0! Oh my GOD. I can die any time now! I started shaking real bad. I was so terrified. I kept saying "How could it be 7.0?" I haven't eaten any differently than I have been for the past 4 years. Then I thought… Oh no, my kidneys must be going bad in a hurry! But that didn't make any sense since my creatinine was only 1.8 and all my other metabolics were normal, except my BUN as usual. I didn't have time to think about it then. My life was on the line and I could die at any moment from the 7.0 Potassium.

Finally, they told me I would need to go to the Emergency Room and have them put me on some inter-venous drug to bring my Potassium level down. My wife and I got ourselves ready to go to the hospital and as bad as I hated going to the hospital, I went because there was no other way to save my life. They said they would let the hospital know I was on my way.

When we arrived, they told us to park by the emergency room thankfully. We rushed in and told them who I was. The girl I talked to after giving another woman my insurance information, said she needed to take my blood pressure. I said "You're not taking my blood pressure! You want to kill me? You take my blood pressure and it's going to scare the f*#king crap out of me and make my blood pressure go through the roof!" She just said "OK. I'll take it and won't tell you what it is." I replied "OK, but don't you dare tell me what it is. It doesn't matter any way."

After that, they led me to one of those little rooms beside the doctor and nurses' station in the ER and had me lay on the table while my wife took a seat next to me. They immediately began to hook all these wires to me to monitor my blood pressure, pulse and my heart. I had to explain to them that even though I have chronic kidney disease, that they needed to realize that I am NOT like all the other kidney patients. I explained that I didn't have any symptoms of chronic kidney disease besides high blood pressure and elevated BUN and creatinine. Well, that is, besides the 7.0 Potassium level I rushed to the ER about. I laid there on the patient table the whole 3 hours I was there.

They took blood and urine to test, but were becoming obsessed and distracted by how high my blood pressure was. It was about 220/120 when I first came in. But the first time I knew about it, my blood pressure was 188/110. They were obsessed with this, but I wasn't bothered about it at all. Your blood pressure goes way up when you are scared or under stress. And I was BOTH, brother! I had feared my Potassium going up like this for the past FOUR years and now that time had come. So all that fear over those four years took control of me once I was told by the doctor's office that my Potassium was 7.0!

While we were waiting on them to tell me the test results, my wife and I discussed what was going on and tried to figure out why my Potassium was 7.0. After a while I told my wife that if I had to choose, I would say that the test result was wrong somehow; even though I had never had any test results that were wrong. Now if my creatinine had've been 2.9 or 3.0, I would've known my kidneys were getting worse and that was the problem. As I laid there, these young nurses kept coming in the room for various reasons.

When one of them asked me for my urine sample I said "Hey, couldn't we have some dinner BEFORE you ask me for my urine?" She got the joke and laughed and smiled as she left the room. When she came back, I asked how long it would be before my test results come back? She said about 45 minutes. They started in on my blood pressure again and gave me 0.2mg Clonidine for it to put under my tongue, as a faster way into my blood stream.

One time when she came in the room asking about my health problems, I looked at her and said "I became the only kidney patient in this area to ever get better. I had to do it myself. Doctors have no cures." She looked at me real funny and said "What?" I said "doctors have no cures", again. She said "Why do you say that?" I said "Well, if doctors have a cure for kidney disease, then tell me what it is right now. I want it!" "And by the way, if you have a cure for diabetes I'll take that right now too just as a precaution." She said "There isn't a cure for kidney disease or diabetes." And I replied "Didn't I just say that?" She smiled and said "Oh, I see why you said that." I said "Yea, because those are the facts. I wish it WASN'T though. I'd much rather be cured than to be right." Shortly after that the ER doctor came in the room.

When he entered my little ER room, the doctor said "Hello Mr. Cooksey. I'm Dr. Allen." I immediately said "No you're not. My doctor is Dr. Allen." He then said "I'm Dr. Allen. There are 3 Dr. Allens in town". I just laughed and let it go. He then began to tell me that my blood test came back and my Potassium was just 4.8. I shouted out "I knew it!" And Dr. Allen continued. He said he was real worried about my blood pressure and that I needed to do this and that.

But I really didn't care, since I was only there because of the 7.0 Potassium. I just wanted out of there. I didn't want to go in the first place. But I told Dr. Allen, Robert I think, that he could do whatever he felt he needed to do to satisfy himself as a doctor before I left. So he gave me some more Clonidine to put under my tongue. I laid there impatiently for about an hour and finally told a nurse that if they didn't take all those wires and IV off me, I was going to do it myself so I could leave. In about 10 minutes or so, they took all the stuff off me, gave me some orders to follow and let me go.

Now as I was leaving, I started thinking about what had just happened. I rushed to the hospital in fear of my life. Ran up a few thousand dollars in medical bills. And did so all because of an errant test result! I was as pissed as I was relieved! I called Dr. Pyle at the hospital and discussed the whole event. I told him I was almost scared to death literally and now had a multi-thousand dollar hospital bill, all because of a wrong test result that came from the hospital's lab in the first place. Dr. Pyle was once again the great reasonable man he had always proven himself to be. He said he would see to it that I didn't get a bill for any of this. I talked to him about what had caused the false test result and how it might be prevented in the future, as well as coming up with some type of protocol to handle this situation in the future.

Dr. Pyle wanted the same thing and said he would get something done about this for the future. I told Dr. Pyle that if I ever have a weird test result like that again, I would ignore it temporarily and go straight back to the doctor's office to give blood for another test. Then, and only then, would I accept the results as valid. He said that was a great idea. I thanked Dr. Pyle and said good bye. I never got a bill. And that brings us to the end of the story up to now.

I went back to the doctor on February 17, 2011 and will be going back in June for my next blood tests. But as far as being scared or worried about my kidneys getting worse and having a relapse or worrying about anything bad happening to me medically, that is pretty much all behind me. I stopped worrying about of dying of chronic kidney disease.

There are some things of importance I didn't get to while I was writing this chapter and going through my incredible journey with the medical profession and through the long line of poisons saturating our food, drinks and water supplies. **To learn about that, read chapters 5, 6 & 7 about Poisons in Your Food, Drinks and Water. Use the information in those chapters to guide you in greatly reducing the amount of poisons in your current diet.**

One other thing I did that really helped my kidneys was to take a product called Kidney Well; which is called Kidney Well II now. You can get this product at www.getwellnatural.com. I try to use it at least every 3 months. A bottle of Kidney Well runs about $60. And every time I ordered Kidney Well I also ordered Alisma. Kidney Well II is made up of 7 herbs: Poria, Alisma, Rehmannia, Ganoderma, Astragalus, Cyperus and Dioscorea in very specific ratios and concentrations that have shown very positive effects for chronic kidney diseases. To me it seems like a strong kidney detox/cleanser. It sure has had a positive effect on my kidneys; especially in lowering my creatinine and BUN and metabolism of Potassium. But with the price being about $10 daily to take it, I can only afford to take it about every 2-3 months.

That investment will certainly do you some real good and far more for your money than what any doctor can do for you. If you hadn't realized it yet... no doctor has ever done a thing to help my kidneys get better; except for Dr. Henry Allen and Dr. David Moskowitz. It's all been about my blood pressure. That's the only help I got from them besides the lab results.

At my first visit to a doctor in 25 years in October 2006, one of the tests they did was an EKG. It had revealed that I also had some heart problems. The main one was that I had an enlarged heart. That is what was causing me to be short of breath quite often. Even when our band was practicing I had to stop in the middle of some songs because I was having too much trouble breathing.

I was told it would most likely only get worse and that it might get a little better if I was lucky. Holy crap! Was I shocked at that information! But once I felt I had my creatinine under control after doing so for 3 years, I asked Dr. Allen to do another EKG. I drove about 15 miles to another office of White River Rural Health and had the EKG done.

I asked for this because of how my blood pressure was always high any time anyone in the medical profession took it. An EKG would show that I had an enlarged heart if my blood pressure had been high for most or a lot of the time. Dr. Allen told me my EKG was "good". I asked if that was good, real good, or just OK. He said it was really good and that I didn't have any heart problems, including no enlarged heart. I was quite relieved at that. And when I went to the ER for that false Potassium test result, they did another EKG. That was about 10 months after the one I just told you about; my second EKG. Dr. Allen said it was even better than the one 10 months earlier! Again, I was super satisfied and excited to know I had been doing a great job of controlling my blood pressure and curing my enlarged heart condition. You might ask "How did you do that?"

What I CAN tell you is this... I made a habit of taking Co-Q10, Magnesium and Fish oil. Co-Q10 helps make your veins and arteries more elastic. So when high blood pressure exerts higher pressure within your circulatory system, your veins and arteries are much less likely to tear or explode; thus causing a stroke or a heart attack. Also, Magnesium not only cures and prevents bladder stones, kidney stones and bone spurs, it causes your heart to relax. Calcium causes your heart to contract, while Magnesium causes your heart to relax. This combined activity is known as your pulse or heartbeat. Uh huh! So if you've got heart arrhythmia or any other problems concerning any abnormalities in your heart beat, Magnesium may very well cure that problem for you.

The Fish oil allows your blood to flow more smoothly and efficiently throughout your body, as well as oiling those arthritic joints and giving you a heaping helping dose of Omega-3. I recommend 250mg Magnesium and 1000mg Fish oil most days for everyone. I have yet to have anyone tell me where they're getting their proper daily dose of Magnesium, and are also hard pressed to tell me where they are getting any Omega-3! So it's almost certain that you are deficient in both Omega-3 and Magnesium.

Some Important Facts about all this – I touched on what I was doing from about December 2006 through present day, all the times I was going to the doctor just like all of you do. What I was doing the whole time was all the things I told you in chapters 5, 6 & 7 to limit, eliminate and avoid the saturation of poisons in our food, drinks and water supply. Ah Ha! Those chapters were about what I was doing habitually and obsessively in those first few years.

Then in this chapter I have been telling you about my difficult experiences with those in the medical profession, as I was learning to do the very things I told you about in those earlier chapters. I didn't want to inject a bunch of details about how I was always busy working on limiting my intake of poisons every or most steps of my story with the medical profession.

So I got those details out of the way in those first few chapters. It doesn't matter what doctor's visit I talked about or time of the day, week, month or year, I was always working to keep the poisons OUT of my body, keep eating healthy and drinking that awesome, life-giving PURE WATER from our fluoride water filter. The fluoride water filter was the first thing we bought to begin our campaign to reduce the large amounts of poisons we were ingesting.

The shower filter was the second thing we did. Oh what tremendous assets both of those babies are for your health. After all, your body IS... 80% water! And do I have to tell you that your body is NOT 80% water plus fluoride plus chlorine!?! Your body is 80% water. So take my advice. Get those water filters first! Every time I feel bad or some discomfort, an upset stomach, tired, puny or the likes, I go get my water jug or bottle and start drinking down that awesome PURE WATER! It never fails to help. I cannot even imagine NOT having a fluoride water filter. I can't believe I never thought it was important to have one, much less have a shower filter too!

How many of you realized that during this entire chapter of telling you my experiences with the medical profession, that I never got any help for

my kidneys from doctors and the medical profession? The one and only exception to that was Dr. David Moskowitz's treatment.

From day one, the doctors did nothing to help my kidneys. See, your kidneys are responsible for many things for your body. Removing poisons is just one of those tasks. So with all the saturation of poisons in everything, your kidneys get overloaded and become soaked with the excess poisons. Your kidneys turn to mush and begin to fail. Of course, I didn't know this before I had chronic kidney disease. With 30 million adults in the US with chronic kidney disease, you'd think someone would care about a cure. I sure do.

So I did what I believed COULD help my kidneys from early 2007, without having anyone to tell me IF what I was doing was going to help my kidneys. No one COULD. No one had ever gotten better at the hands of this country's doctors and medical profession. But regardless of how willfully incompetent doctors are about curing diseases, I still had to find a way to cure myself or at least get better. And while I was doing everything to help my kidneys, I got some near miraculous surprises:

I cured myself of arthritis – What do I mean exactly? I had arthritis for at least 20 years. Most of that time I would have swollen painful joints 4 or 5 days every week. But after going cold turkey on the sodas and fruit juices for a few months, I noticed I wasn't hardly getting any swollen, painful joints. I had been taking Glucosamine a lot. But when I started taking Fish oil regularly at that time, those swollen, painful red joints disappeared. And to this day, I still haven't had any arthritis. I'm going on seven years without arthritis. Doctors say arthritis is NOT curable. I cured myself merely by taking Magnesium, Fish oil and Vitamin C. Can you GUESS if I believe that! I am so thankful that I don't!

I cured myself of heartburn, acid reflux – What do I mean exactly? I had acid reflux for at least 20 years too. I had heartburn pretty much all the time. I had heartburn at least 4 or 5 times a day that I HAD to take some TUMS for immediately! I got to where I would take those little ant-acid tablets to get some relief. You take those to prevent heartburn. But even though I took them every day, I still had heartburn, but not as much. I still had heartburn daily. But while I was concentrating on finding something that would help my kidneys, my heartburn came to an end. I took apple cider vinegar for some bouts of heartburn for a few months after starting the crusade to avoid the poisons in our food, drinks and water. But after that my heartburn went away.

I cured myself of headaches – What do I mean exactly? For the past 20 years or so I have had headaches. I didn't have hardly any when I was a kid or teenager that I can remember. But into my early twenties, I started getting headaches every once and awhile. As the years have gone by I just accepted that headaches were normal. Everyone gets them. Some people MORE. Some people LESS. But just a few months into the start of my poison crusade, just like the arthritis and heartburn, the headaches faded away. I was so busy trying to save my own life, that I was only concerned about helping my kidneys get better so I didn't have to die or start dialysis in 2008. I never did anything with the intent of curing anything besides chronic kidney disease! I was really surprised at being cured of all this. But hey, there's more!

I cured myself of dandruff – I thought only Head and Shoulders cured dandruff! No, I don't think they make that claim. But dandruff is a common thing too. I use to have dandruff flakes on the shoulders of my shirts all the time. I could shake or brush my hair and watch the flakes fly in the air. I noticed that about other people too, but never said anything to anyone; since dandruff was so common. But barely two months passed after we got our shower filter and my dandruff was all but gone completely!

I look back and say "Of course you have dandruff. You're soaking your scalp with that chlorinated water that destroys the oils in your skin, scalp and hair!" It's pretty much unavoidable unless you use a shower filter. And doing that also cured me of the red, itchy spots on my body I always got and were irritated every time I took a shower. This also cured my wife of the same thing and dandruff. Just think of how much money we've saved with the greatly lower use of all the dandruff shampoos and skin lotions?

We always thought dandruff was normal and never could find anything to stop those red, itchy places on our bodies! No one told me these things. I learned them and proved them by personal experiences.

I cured myself of gout – I didn't have gout for 20 years daily like the other diseases and conditions I just mentioned. I had one gout attack around 2000 and didn't have another one until late 2007. It lasted for about two weeks, then went away without me doing anything specifically about gout. Dr. Henry Allen gave me medication to take if I thought I was getting gout again.

I used those pills once right after that two month episode with gout in September and October of 2009. Then took one pill on two future occasions shortly after that, but never developed gout again. Getting back on the high fructose corn syrup brought me two months of gout every day all day. But once I got back off the high fructose corn syrup and drank baking soda water, the gout went away and stayed away. Boy am I glad. It was this that sealed the deal for eternity about high fructose corn syrup being the addicting poison that it is.

The thing that finally ended my gout was me adding pH drops to my drinking water and drinking baking soda and water. I got the pH drops off Ebay. A two months' supply is only about $8. Baking soda is 89¢ for a 1-lb. box; making it medicinal gold. All disease has to have an acidic environment to exist. So by drinking highly alkaline water, water with baking soda or pH drops, you begin to neutralize the acid that causes all disease. This is the first step you wanna take when you have any disease; especially chronic "incurable" disease.

One great fact that you must learn is that these corporations put these poisons in their products mainly to addict you to their products and turn you into a robot consumer. What I mean by robot consumer is that you buy these poison saturated products and stuff them down your throat and never consider what you're doing - poisoning yourself and creating sickness inside your body. Is THIS what you really want to do? I don't really think so.

So why do you do it again and again, day after week after month, year in year out? It's because your mind has a craving for those poisons. You ate some food item saturated with poisons and even though it didn't nourish your body as real food does, that food or drink gave your body sensations as those poisons were damaging your body. I hope I have repeated these facts enough.

This is where you gain the victory over those poisons - in your mind; as you are eating or drinking these poison saturated foods and drinks. Do the food or drinks nourish you, or are you eating and drinking those products because you have a craving for them in your head? I talked about this earlier, about using this information to see if you like whole milk or are addicted to the drugs and chemicals in the milk's fat. I also did this with tea.

I cured myself of bleeding gums – This was another big surprise to me. My gums had been bleeding a lot for about 15-20 years prior to my kidneys failing. It got to where every time I brushed my teeth, my gums would start bleeding in front and then in other places. That always turned my sudsy white toothpaste into pink sudsy toothpaste every time. I lost some teeth from this too. And all this time I was brushing my teeth 6 or 7 times every day. I brushed after I ate or drank anything. My gums bled every time in spite of my excess brushing habit.

But just like the heartburn, headaches, arthritis and other chronic conditions I had for up to twenty years had faded away during the first six months of my poison elimination crusade, my gums stopped bleeding. They stopped bleeding for a few months before I was willing to believe my gums might not bleed again. And over the years since they first stopped bleeding in 2007, my gums haven't bled at all from brushing. The only time my gums bleed now is when I puncture them or cut them with a dental pick. You know, one of those hook shaped metal tooth picks on a 6-inch plastic stick/handle. My gums have firmed up and my teeth have too. My gums gave me the visual for what my kidneys must have looked like when they failed… mushy, soft and slowly disintegrating.

I have also cured or all but cured myself of chronic kidney disease. My last blood tests revealed that I am closer than ever.

I also prevented myself from developing diabetes. The doctors were always looking for that and said that almost all patients with chronic kidney disease develop diabetes. No doubt, I teetered on the edge of diabetes sometimes, but did specific things to try and prevent that. If you read the information on how to cure diabetes, you may be surprised at what I learned to help my pancreas to prevent diabetes.

I also cured myself of other conditions like internal intestinal bleeding and bladder stones which I had for several years back in the mid 90's.

But what I have achieved with my kidneys makes me a pioneer in curing chronic kidney disease. I know I could have done a better job and still can. But I was too busy DOING all these things to see IF and WHAT helped, if anything. So I had to have it proven to me for an extended period of time before I could talk about any of this being a cure.

Hey, it might have just been a normal break from headaches, heartburn and/or arthritis. No one told me any of this would cure anyone. And I searched the INTERNET and quizzed every nurse and doctor I've ever come into contact with about any cures for these things! Or maybe there's a powerful conspiracy against just ME, to make sure I am the ONLY one who never gets to hear these alleged "cures" the rest of you already know? Let me know IF you have any proof of that! LOL I would like to save your life and have you avoid most sickness and suffering. But only YOU can do that for yourself and your family. **This book gives you the information to guide you in doing just that.**

I went ahead and wrote this book so that people could prevent all these diseases and cure them too. I am not saying I have the complete story on cures and preventions. But I do know I am telling you the most important and most powerful things to do AND the most important things NOT to do, in order to change your health in the most positive ways you never thought possible.

I am not some author who came up with a new subject for my next book I wish to market! I am the guy who became the only person in this country that got better after being diagnosed with chronic kidney disease; and did so by doing things I had to learn and prove in order to save my own life. These are my credentials. This is my proof of how I proved I could do what this country's modern medical profession could not and/or would not do... help a person with chronic kidney disease(CKD) get better! So even if you only have CKD caused by hypertension, doing what I set forth in this book will delay dialysis for years and very possibly avoid dialysis altogether.

Even if I started getting worse now, I wouldn't need dialysis until early 2017; NINE YEARS after doctors said I would be on dialysis. So far I've saved nearly $500,000 in medical bills. That's about $50,000 in medical bills and the $100,000 a year for dialysis. Now if this idea catches on, the health-care crisis will end real fast! The millions of bankruptcies over medical bills would end and your suffering would greatly diminish. The food companies won't change until you refuse to buy their poisons. And the way you stop buying their poisons is by reading the labels while you're in the grocery store and never putting that garbage in your basket to bring it home.

For now, you all have to do this for yourselves, since We the People have no government to do this for us. FDA approved safe - still killing us by the tens of thousands yearly, because the concept of poisons being bad hinders corporate profits. **You won't knock the chip off my shoulder! It got glued on when they tried to poison me to death.**

I had set out to do something to try and help my kidneys get better so I could avoid dialysis or at least delay dialysis and maybe save my life. I never had any intention of writing a book about any of this. I also never set out to cure myself of anything but chronic kidney disease. After all, doctors said I would be dead no later than 2009 unless I got a successful kidney transplant. And that was only a possibility! No doctors had done anything to help my kidneys. So it was all up to me to help myself if I was going to get any help for my kidneys.

Now what is so troubling about doctors is that I went to them for help and a cure. But even though I went to the doctor again and again and again, I never got one bit of help for my kidneys! **How the heck does anyone expect doctors to help them when doctors won't even as much as TRY to do anything to help your kidneys when you are diagnosed with chronic kidney disease!**

All they do is preach death and dialysis while they hold your hand and lead you to your grave without any hope or cure; in order to maximize their income. And do so without any regard for your life or your health. This willful incompetence is THE WAY of the medical profession when it comes to sickness and disease. I wish it was not true. But it is.

What I did to help my kidneys has proven to be unknown among doctors and the medical profession. You can NOT learn how to get better with chronic kidney disease from doctors. You can't get a cure for arthritis, headaches, acid reflux, gout, diabetes or even the common cold from the medical profession. All my help for my kidneys came from myself. And I proved that what I had done actually worked and did so with proof that no doctor has denied.

I'm alive right now because of what I learned since 2007. This is my story about how I saved my own life and cured myself. And if you want to do the same, this book is your only hope. And you are hearing from the horse's mouth, how the horse saved his own life, doing the things that the horse had to learn and prove while waiting to die, in order for the horse to save his own life.

And I did it! So maybe you are one of those who loses his car keys and looks on the TV and doesn't find them and then does what no one is doing about their own health and lives… you look elsewhere until you find those keys.

- **So, as the doctors give you NO CURES when you go to them.**
- **Just LOOK ELSEWHERE for a cure and you'll find it!**
- **That is how I found a cure for my chronic kidney disease.**
- **That is how I found the cure for ALL my chronic diseases.**
- **And that is how I found the cure/cures for ALL disease, except some of the ones caused by viruses and germs.**

13 - Helping your Dogs and other Pets

I wish I had known what I know today back when my dogs had died, at various times, of conditions that could have been easily avoided. I watched my little Cockapoo suffer with bladder stones for years. She had peed out a dozen or so white bladder stones that I saw with my own eyes. When she was 12 years old, almost 13, she had bladder surgery to remove a stone. Now this stone was the size of a golf ball. The vet said it was the largest stone they had ever removed from a dog of any size. And at the end of her days six years later, at age 18, she died from her spine freezing up with calcium deposits, aka bone spurs. I never ran across anything to help her. We took her to the Vet to get all the help they could give her. So I had already asked lots of people if they knew how to prevent or help dogs in that condition.

Then we had a Great Dane to live to age 13 and the same thing happened to him. We fed him far better food than all previous dogs; meaning, we didn't feed the Great Dane much dog food. We got him eating organic broccoli and other fresh organic vegetables and fruit. But still, the same thing happened to him with his spine freezing up. He didn't have any sick days his entire life until that last year of his life.

I was overwhelmed with determination to solve this problem for dogs. And it's this determination to stop dogs from this suffering and having to die from this that brought me to the solution. What happened with my Cockapoo that lived 18 years was the information I used to cure myself of "incurable" bladder stones. What I learned was a possible solution for her bladder stones is the exact solution I used to cure myself of "incurable" bladder stones.

You see, Magnesium dissolves calcium in your body, so that calcium can be used by your body. If you do not have enough Magnesium, those stray particles of calcium bind to toxins, aka free radicals, to form those prickly little bladder stones. The same scientific principle is also true about other calcium deposits in your body known as kidney stones and bone spurs.

So when I had that fourth bladder stone attack, I put that very information to the test to see IF it would work or help at all. I had endured 2 attacks that lasted for 3 or 4 days by myself; not knowing what it was, or how long it would last. The third attack I went to the hospital for a $1000+ ER bill and just avoided a $5000 hospital bill. That was only because I refused to check in to the hospital for a few days. When the fourth attack came, I thought of what I had learned about my dog's bladder stones. I took two 250mg Magnesium oxide tablets about 20-30 minutes into the attack, and within 45 minutes the attack was over.

I used a screened strainer, they had given me at the hospital, to pee through the rest of the day, but there was never any trace of a stone or debris in it. So it made sense that the Magnesium had dissolved the calcium in a small stone in me and ended the pain and discomfort completely. To be honest, I wasn't

100% positive at first. But as over 15 years have gone by without another bladder stone attack, I have taken Magnesium regularly. It's proven science.

I got to test my knowledge on this with our present dog just after she turned 6 years old. I had taken what I learned in my efforts to stop this common problem plaguing dogs and came to my own conclusion as to what might prevent this problem in dogs. I had scheduled that very solution to begin for our present dog at age 7. But as our present dog turned 6, a few months after that her behavior began to change. She no longer wanted to jump up on the bed a dozen times a day. She didn't want to stand on her back legs and hug us with her front legs and didn't even want to stand up the same way and drink out of the bathroom sink faucet! We thought she would get over it at first.

But about 4 or 5 months into this behavior I decided to start her on my solution immediately, instead of waiting until age 7. A few weeks after I got her started on my solution, our dog started doing the things she had always done, once again. She never shows any sign of that problem anymore. It's been several years now. That is a complete turnaround on that problem plaguing most older dogs - lack of Omega-3 and Magnesium - in just 3 or 4 weeks.

That was my planned solution. 1000mg Fish oil and 250mg Magnesium twice a day for 10-14 days. Then once a day for the next 2-3 months. Then a maintenance dose once a day every few days or at least twice a week, from now on. Start your dogs on the maintenance dose at least by age 6.

Getting that water filter for yourself will also help the health of your pets too. Your pets are drinking that same chlorinated, fluoridated water you have been drinking. The chlorine in that water kills the bacteria in an animal's stomach and intestines just the same as it does inside you. Your pets live a much shorter life than you do. So giving your pets pure water to drink will go a long ways toward your pets' health and extending their lives.

Killing fleas – I can't believe I spent my whole life fighting fleas. I have tried everything to get rid of fleas. Sometimes we would be rid of fleas for a few months, only to have fleas again. I would spread Diazinon on the yard where we let our dogs out. It worked very well too. Having that determination to get rid of fleas finally led me to the ultimate solution! We got some Twenty Mule Team borax at Wal-Mart and spread it on all our carpet using a 4 inch tea strainer. We were to vacuum it up after 24 hours and that's what we did.

When I vacuumed the first room, I looked in the clear bin on our Dyson vacuum cleaner that collects all the dirt and debris vacuumed up and could see fleas jumping around in the white borax powder. There were quite a few dead ones too. My wife and I decided to spread borax on the carpet in another room and then walked on it with our bare feet and we saw fleas hopping on our feet. It was very odd, but also very clear that those fleas wanted to get away from that borax! So we left the borax on for just 2-3 hours in the rest of the rooms in our house. We didn't want the fleas to get a chance to come back, so we did the whole house again about 2 weeks later. That was in the summer of 2005. We haven't seen a flea since. Well, we did pick a flea off our dog on occasion. But that's all! And our cats haven't had any fleas either. No ticks also.

Before I used the borax, I had found a great way to kill fleas off my dogs. What you do is give your dog a bath just like you normally do. Then, once you have rinsed off the soap, do this. Make about a quart of a mixture of 3 parts water, 1 part apple cider vinegar and pour this down the back of your dog's neck to his tail. Do your best to rub it into their hair. Not only will this mixture kill all the fleas, it will bring great relief to your pets' red itching skin. These red itchy places, where your dog's hair falls off or gets thin, are caused by fungus that fleas spread through biting your pets' flesh, and flea poop. And since apple cider vinegar is an alkalizing substance, it neutralizes that acidic fungus.

When we started doing this for our dog, her rear end and back next to her tail was bare. Within 3-4 weeks of using the apple cider vinegar on her, the hair had all grown back. I was really shocked. We had spent lots of money on getting her shots at the vet for this, as well as all the different high priced dog shampoos we had tried on her. And we end up curing her with a dollar's worth of apple cider vinegar! That just goes back to what I said at the very first of this book....... you can afford the cures, but not the treatments.

Now we use baking soda water to stop those acidic flea bite areas on our dog. Use at the rate of 1 teaspoon per quart of water for a final rinse. We alternate between the ACV and baking soda as an overall solution. Right now we are trying to get our pets to drink some baking soda water to see if they need excess acid neutralized to improve their health.

In this case it was hundreds of dollars for treatment, but only ONE DOLLAR for a cure. It made me feel like an idiot at first. But getting THE CURE for my dog is very uplifting. It's great never seeing her suffer like she did all summer, every summer at the first of her life. And hey, the Twenty Mule Team borax was only about $3 too. $1 to cure my dog's red itchy bald spots. $3 to rid our dogs, cats and house of fleas! This tip alone is worth the cost of this book!

When buying dog food you have a lot of choices. Not much dog food is very healthy. The main thing to look for is inside the bag. See how many grease spots there are inside the bag of dog food. The more grease and oil spots there are on the inside of the bag, the worse the food quality is. Find a bag of dog food that doesn't have any oily spots inside the bag or only a very few. Then stick with that specific dog food. You want to try and avoid foods with meat by products and additives like BHA and BHT. Avoid dog foods with corn, wheat or soy if you can.

To compare a healthy dog food like BLUE dog food to most popular brands go to this web page: http://bluebuffalo.com/dog-food-comparison/test-results.

There's another organic dog food called Eukanuba. I have fed it to my dog and my cats before. I even caught my cats eating it out of the dog food bowl.

But both of these dog foods are around $50 per 25lb bag dry. You can find out about Eukanuba on their site here: http://www.eukanuba.com/en-US.

We actually feed our dog the same food that we eat. Our dog and cats gather around the table for just about every meal. Or I should say, they stick to our sides even when we're eating. Hehe! Our dog always gets what's left after each meal. But our cats will only eat fish, chicken and turkey. We have gotten them to eat broccoli and brown rice sometimes too. We put some Purina Beneful out for our dog to eat too. But a 25lb bag of Beneful lasts at least 6 months; since most food our dog eats is the same food we eat.

Our dogs have always eaten food from our organic gardens. We started feeding them fresh produce when they were young pups about 6 months old. They love broccoli and cheese, tomatoes, garden vegetable soup and more. Our dogs also eat the produce we buy at the grocery stores, such as grapes, strawberries, watermelon, kiwi fruit, bananas and other fresh fruit, but not a lot of vegetables. It's easy to concentrate on feeding fresh produce to your dog when they are sick or hurt, as a big part of the healing process. But I've never been able to do that for cats. Don't feed a dog too many grapes.

When it comes to cats, I'm pretty much lost as to how to help them and if they will even let me help them. It's usually just take them to the vet or do nothing. And that is hard for me to do. One very serious problem that kills lots of cats is a urinary tract infection. This problem will kill your cat in just a few days; 3 – 4 days many times. So it's tragic many times. If your cat's behavior suddenly changes and stays that way more than a day, you should pay close attention to your cat for any signs of sickness.

When a cat has a urinary tract infection, they will start pissing outside of the litter box. One of our cats came within a few hours of dying from a urinary tract infection. And that is where we woke up about this sad fact. This problem affects male cats more often than female cats. The reason is obvious. A male cat has a narrow penis he has to pee out of and this restricts the flow of urine more than in female cats. Once the food your cat has been eating causes grit to form in the bladder, it begins to restrict the urinal tract as it increases and builds. This backs the urine back into the bladder and kidneys and organ failure sets in. Death comes within a few hours without medical attention.

The vet has to run a tube through the cat's urinary tract to open it up so urine can flow out. This takes about 3 days. The bill for this runs at least $500 and your cat almost dies. So you have to take this problem seriously if you love your cats. There's a few things you can do to help.

Buy urinary tract formula cat food like: Purina One Urinary Tract Formula or Hill's Multicare Feline Bladder Health

Feeding your cat Hill's canned version of their Feline Bladder Health cat food will help even better than the dry version of the same cat food; because of the moisture canned food adds to your cat's body. We feed our cats these cat foods, along with the fish, chicken and turkey they eat out of our human food. Cats tend to puke if you feed them salty foods like hot dogs, ham, bologna and other sliced lunch and deli meats. And our two house cats have never been sick, except for the one that had this urinary tract infection and obstruction after he turned 8 years old.

Don't ever punish your cat if he/she pisses outside the litter box. Sure you don't like to clean it up or smell it. But..... be thankful to know the warning signs of real health problems in your cats. Punishing your pet robs you of the chance to save your pet. Instead of seeing their SUDDEN bad behavior as a sign something is wrong, you fool yourself into believing you have solved the problem by punishing them.

And keep an eye on them until they are back to normal. If your cat stops pissing for 24 hours, you need to get your cat to the vet immediately. You can ask a veterinarian about any of these facts. I told you because I don't want your cats to die or you only learning all this after the fact.

What we finally did for our cats was feed them yogurt. We knew that the two beneficial bacteria in yogurt aid in the health of our stomach. But we weren't sure if that would help cats. But after we switched our cats to Hill's Urinary Tract Formula dry food, our two indoor cats kept throwing up. The Hill's does prevent that grit in a cat's urinary tract that stops up their male pee hole and will kill cats in 3 or 4 days. But it didn't do hardly a thing for the regular throwing up.

Now some of the throwing up is from hair cats ingest licking themselves and each other. But we felt it was more than that. So we applied a proven scientific principle and started feeding them some yogurt. But since all store bought yogurt contains twice as much sugar as yogurt, we weren't sure if it would do any good. But even with all that sugar, it did help.

We looked and looked for plain yogurt but could barely ever find any. So I finally used some of that sugary yogurt and made my own like I use to do. And once we started feeding them the PURE plain yogurt, they both stopped throwing up almost completely. Feed them as much yogurt as they will eat. Try about a tablespoon per cat a few times a day. Sprinkle a few bits of their dry cat food on the yogurt to get them eating the yogurt. It's such a relief to see all this improvement in our cats' health. And even more so now that we have seen this sustained in our cats since the middle of 2011.

Now, just a few more brief tips to help your pets –

- **We give our dog 1000mg Vitamin C, 250mg Magnesium and 1200mg Fish oil every few days. Do this once your dog turns 6 and once a week the first 6 years**
- **Don't use medicated or flea shampoos – Use organic soap such as Dr. Bonner's soap or just use the same shampoo or soap as you use on yourself. Dish detergent also works just fine. And rinse your dog with apple cider vinegar/water mixed – 1 part apple cider vinegar, 3 parts water;**

8-ounces ACV to 24-ounces water to kill all fleas and alkalize your dog's skin to ease and cure the balding red spots flea allergies cause most dogs.

- Never give your cat aspirin, unless your veterinarian tells you to.
- Never feed your dog chocolate. It can kill a dog.
- Never allow your dog to eat anything with the sweetener Xylitol, such as low calorie gum or Xylitol mints. Consuming Xylitol can kill a dog.
- Never leave your dog tied in the sun or without water.
- Never beat or whip your pets. Dogs and cats respond to love; dogs more so than cats. Whipping them only causes them to think you're mean and makes the animal mean. Scolding your pets verbally is enough.
- Take the time and effort to make sure your pets eat healthy food and drink the purest water possible. This goes a very long way in helping your pets live longer and healthier lives.
- And most of all, love them unconditionally just like they do you! I've always used active love to create the relationships between all my pets and myself. Sure they irritate me. Rarely but not too often. But I only think of how much I love them and how bad it will hurt when they're gone. So I let every bit of it go, as it happens. One of my cats will race away from me when I yell at her for doing something bad. Then in one motion, race right back to me. That cat has never been scared of anything. Amazing, but absolutely true. She was born in our house.
- BE the Master. Being the Master isn't confined to just being the boss and the pet obeys the Master. IF..... if you ARE the Master, then BE the Master. The Master knows if his animals are hurting, sick or in need and meets those needs. The Master feeds his animals good wholesome food too. And because of the information I have shared in this chapter, you can afford to BE the Master, regardless of your income.

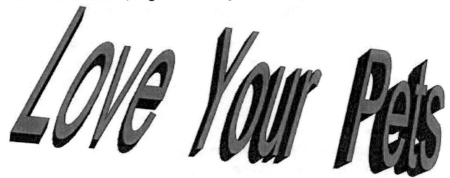

I had 2 Great Danes live to be 13 years old and neither was sick until their final year of life. I had a Cockapoo live to age 18. So I thought you'd like to know some of the things I learned to accomplish that with my dogs. Hope this helps add time to your pets' lives. I wish someone had shared this with me a few decades ago! Yes, oh how I wish!

14 -How to Have an Organic Garden

I started gardening back in 1981. My first year, I gardened pretty much like everyone else did. But when I got to having to use Seven dust and Malathion, I didn't like gardening as well as I thought I would. The thought of being gagged by those poisons just to garden, was pretty frightening. The next year I moved to a house with a much bigger yard and begin looking for ways to kill bugs and fungus and fertilize that were not chemicals. Nobody talked much about organic gardening back then.

And for at least a decade, people laughed at my organic gardening ways. It was mostly because they had used nothing but chemicals on their gardens. But the one thing that finally shut them up and changed their tune to me, was the results I was getting in my garden.

Plenty of people would drive by and yell out things like "Your garden looks great!" and "You've got the best garden in the county" or "You've got the best garden in town" and other nice compliments. People would stop and tell me the same things and wanted to know what my secret was. That was rewarding and funny because of all the ones who had turned their noses at what I was doing.

Right from the start of my organic gardening days, I was adding organic material to the soil. I used anything I could get, like horse manure, cow manure, hay, wheat straw, shredded paper, rice hulls and a few others. But instead of going into a long drawn out story about organic gardening tips and so on, let me get right to the information you must have and learn in order to achieve an organic garden.

I am not really going to tell you HOW to garden. I am telling you how to make your gardening Organic. And to do that you have to have fertilizer, fungicide and pesticides. Here are some organic alternatives for those chemical products. These are all things I use.

- **Fungicide – Use Liquid Copper, Liquid Sulfur, baking soda or hydrated lime.**
- **Pesticides – Use Bt for worms & Rotenone for hard shell insects**
- **Fertilizers – Use liquid kelp, fish emulsion and Spray N Grow**

You can get all these organic products from:

Spray-N-Grow at: http://www.spray-n-growgardening.com

And Gardens Alive at: http://www.gardensalive.com

The one product I can't do without is Spray-N-Grow. I've never seen anything that achieves the results that Spray-N-Grow gives. It's not actually a fertilizer, but you will think it is. Spray-N-Grow has 40 different nutrients, which causes your plants to be more healthy, produce more flowers and produce, resist bugs and make your produce sweeter.

I spray the plants every few days when they are small. Then spray them about every 10-14 days or so. It's the most efficient way to use it. Put a few drops of liquid dish soap as a "wetting agent" to help the solution stick to the surfaces of the plant.

Fish emulsion stinks, but is a good fertilizer. Giving your plants more than the usual Phosphorous, Nitrogen and Potassium makes plants significantly more healthy. Plants need far more nutrients than that. And using Spray-N-Grow, fish emulsion and liquid kelp/seaweed does exactly that. They all give your plants the wide array of nutrients they need.

Just as some diseases are caused by lack of nutrients, your garden plants will be far less damaged by bugs and disease. They will also be far more healthy than using only Potassium, Phosphorous and Nitrogen.

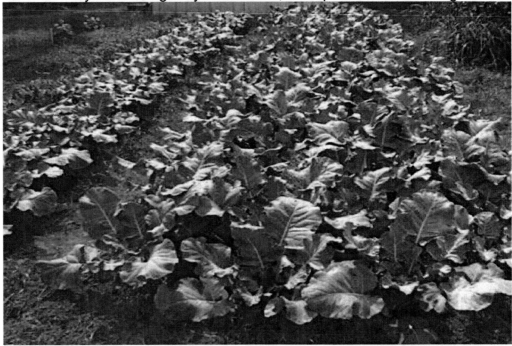

Another good tip is to plant your garden plants in beds of 3 to 4 staggered rows. I take a piece of cardboard and draw a triangle on the cardboard with all sides being 15 inches long. Then I cut the triangle shape out of the piece of cardboard and cut the points off each of the 3 triangle points. You try to cut a round cut for these 3 points.

So you use a string and stakes to stretch the string the length of the row you want, then shove the stakes in the ground. Take the triangle piece of cut out cardboard and lay it with the bottom in line with the string, with the top point of the triangle headed into the bed.

Plant a plant at each side of the triangle in the row. Then plant a plant at the top of the triangle. Move the triangle to the side of the last plant planted in the first row and repeat this process again and again. You will end up with row 1 planted with plants 15 inches apart, and the second row will be about 13 inches from the first row, with the 2nd row of plants staggered from the first row.

This allows you to use your garden space in the most efficient way and allows the plants to cover the entire garden space as they grow. This also saves a lot of time with spraying, conserves water and the roots from the plants aerate the soil for the plants around each other. (Picture above shows part of my garden planted using an 18-inch triangle, the same way as the 15-inch triangle. Bed on the left is 2 rows broccoli and 2 rows tomatoes in one bed.)

Gardeners usually just plant one straight row, then have 3-4 feet in between rows. That style is for field planting with tractors, not for home gardens! The idea is to have as much of your garden covered by plants as you possibly can, while making sure you leave room to walk in your garden to care for it properly.

A perfect idea would be to have long beds about 6-feet wide with 3-foot tall sides all around with rot resistant wood. Fill that with sphagnum peat moss, Perlite, top soil, sand and about 25% other organic materials. These raised beds will grow things extremely well. Just add an irrigation system of some sort; even soaker hoses made with recycled tires. Bury them about 3-inches deep; same as you would for plastic pipe systems.

I don't mind admitting that I do use some 13-13-13 fertilizer a little. And I also use Miracle-Gro. I mix Miracle-Gro in with the liquid seaweed and fish emulsion and spray it all at once. It's all fertilizer. I don't ever use any other non-organic materials besides the 13-13-13 and Miracle-Gro.

You can also kill soft shelled insects by just spraying dish detergent mixed with water. Kill hard shelled insects with Rotenone and Pyrethrum. www.groworganic.com is another good place to find these.

As for fungicides, since fungus and molds are acidic, we have been using baking soda as a fungicide. I knew it worked in principle, but was not sure until I tried it on some broccoli seedlings. They went limp and my wife couldn't figure out what to do. So I told her to spray them with baking soda – 1 teaspoon per 40 ounces water and they came back to life! So that was all the proof we needed to switch to baking soda.

Since lime is also highly alkaline, you can also use hydrated lime as a fungicide. I have friends who told me about hydrated lime when I was telling them about the baking soda. We all use lime to raise the pH of the soil and provide calcium, manganese and magnesium. So using hydrated lime as a fungicide should be acceptable to most of you already.

So, just go on gardening the way you always have. But buy the Organic versions of pesticides, fungicides and fertilizers as I told you in this chapter. And work on adding organic materials to your soil. Within a few years you will have good rich soil, your garden will be much more healthy and vigorous and you'll enjoy nothing but the freshest, highest quality, poison free produce you use to could only imagine!

You know what's in it, because YOU are the one who gave every plant the ingredients to grow. Or in this case we should say that you are the one who did NOT put the poisons in the soil and on the plants.

It use to irk me to no end to grow a garden to have the healthiest food possible. Then always be pressured to buy the chemicals to poison it, because of how you can get the chemicals so many places, but have to hunt for Organic products!

So take the time and grow that garden right – with no poisons added!

My Final Words

I get a lot of satisfaction every time I get to the end of one of my books. That has to do with how hard I work to make sure I get every bit of information that can possibly help you cure yourselves. And at the same time, I follow my long term principles of accurate information and making sure I do not say anything that is wrong or can hurt you. Although the results you get from using the proven science shared in this book will be just as stated, I don't like to get off on all that miracle talk. I wish I could go along with that. Proven science certainly is marvelous, helpful and deeply interesting. I just don't see how I can claim the scientific cures in this book are "miracles". So I never have.

A miracle would come from God, like laying hands on you to cure you or by driving some demons out of you as is the way in the bible. But people just don't relate to miracles this way anymore. So we see things like Goji juice and other single products that are claiming to be "miracle cures". The anti-oxidants in Goji or any product are not enough to cure anyone. I never claim one thing will cure you. And as close a thing I know to making that claim is baking soda. But since no disease is caused by lack of baking soda, there is no way mere baking soda alone COULD cure you. Using it to reverse the acidic state of your body is the single most important thing to do when curing yourself though.

Funny thing is that I cured myself of everything but gout without using baking soda water. I now know that I would have cured myself much faster if I had just had ONE person to tell me to drink baking soda water to reverse the metabolic acidosis which is the foundation of your kidney disease. By soaking our acidic kidneys with high alkaline baking soda water, you neutralize acid in your entire body. Your kidneys do this by creating a more alkaline blood, which flows throughout your body, of course! And cancer or any chronic disease cannot even exist in an alkaline body.

My final words are about reminding you of the importance of what is stated in this book. Baking soda is the most important, followed by pure water and a shower filter. You soak up la whole lot of poisons in the shower and bath tub.

It is the overall total amount of poisons that eventually overtake your body's immune system that creates disease.

This is the reason **this book is not a diet book, but a book about avoiding poisons in your food, drinks and water supplies, as well as our hygiene products like soap, shampoo, deodorants, lotions and such.**

It is poisons that cause at least 80% of all disease. So avoiding those poison saturated products is a **requirement** if you expect to be cured and stay cured. You avoid the poisons, flush your body with clean pure filtered water and shower in it. You drink the baking soda water to reverse your body's diseased acidic state. You take anti-oxidants to remove the poisons in your body which cause all disease. You take Magnesium to get over 300 body metabolisms to occur once again, among other things. Take the Fish or Flax seed oil. Then do as much of the other things that you can.

To avoid the saturation of poisons and to see your way to genuine natural alternatives for products you consume, you need to learn chapters 6 & 7 by heart. Let it become a part of you. That way YOU will always be there to keep those saturation of poisons out of your body and the bodies of your families. The sad thing about this is that poisons have overwhelmed our food and drinks since the mid-1980s. That's when President Reagan refused to help any of our struggling family farmers, so that his buddies could buy all the family farms and thus cease control of the costs, supplies AND content of our food supplies.

And as soon as they did, here comes that hellish death substance called high fructose corn syrup. And quickly, we went from having ZERO products with genetically modified high fructose corn syrup to almost every product in every grocery store containing HFCS! Manipulating people's minds with drugs so that they have abnormal cravings for products soaked with HFCS is not and never has been legal under our Laws. But since it's all about unbridled greed, this illegal behavior is not only tolerated, it is APPROVED and protected by our crony fascist government, of the corporations, by the corporations and for the corporations. It takes a while for this sick crap to sink in, I promise.

But it's all up to YOU to just read labels and avoid their poisons; high fructose corn syrup, any and all other sugars, salts, fats, Trans-fats and so on. And by doing so you will be rewarding yourselves doubly! How? By avoiding their high cost processed products and saving all those high costs of those medical bills you won't be needing. Not to mention, how you get to live much longer and live that life with no disease. So that's at least TRIPLE rewards.

IF I had the attitude of doctors, this book would be priced at around $8000. That would still be a tremendous bargain compared to any health benefits you could ever get from doctors when it comes to curing disease. One of the major principles at work here is that knowledge is Power! How much money did I need to cure my kidney disease? Or heart disease, arthritis or gout? The answer is always - no amount of money will get you cured, because there is NO cure for your chronic disease! But the knowledge in this book brought you cures for your diseases. And it only cost a few dollars!

The truth in this book set me free of all my diseases. That knowledge for you to do the same thing is what I put in this book and tried the best I could to explain it. Just as I told you about not knowing to drink baking soda water and had to learn that AFTER I cured myself of everything but gout, is part of how I am still learning. I'm sure this information could be presented better. But because I am still learning, my knowledge of cures is evolving as it grows. But my principles and proven science I have learned, do not change. They are the foundation on which all other things are discovered and proven.

Realizing that baking soda neutralizes acids is one new law of physics I have put to use personally; all the way from finally knocking my gout out to becoming my toothpaste and deodorant. Not to mention now using it in the garden as a fungicide; killing that acidic state fungus and mold must have to exist on plants. And baking soda will cost you a dollar or two monthly for all that combined.

One thing I am researching now is natural remedies for pain and infections. And as always, I am building on the proven scientific principles I have already learned. It seems that clove oils, cinnamon, colloidal silver, raw honey, bee propolis, chamomile and others can be used for pain and/or infections. And who doesn't wanna know that!

Say your gums get infected so your tooth and maybe jaw hurts bad. What is your only way now? Yep, call the dentist and let those heartless turds tell you they can get you an appointment in 2-3 weeks! So you sit and suffer with bad pain in your face because your only help is the dentist. So we all need a solution to help us at those times. And that is just one example of an area of our health care needs which need natural solutions.

Before doctors abandoned all cures and all natural medicines starting in the 1940s, all of our medicines were natural medicines. There were no prescription drugs before 1939. Everything the medical profession and doctors do was invented by them! So all I have really done is go back to the way it ALWAYS was until the past 75 years or so and proceed! Then learning to recognize the saturation of disease causing poisons in products is a new requirement for being cured that has not existed before the mid-1980s. This is what sets this and all my books apart from all others. So if you gotta put a label on ME, it would be pro-cure, not anti-doctor or anti-medical profession or anti anything. The one thing I am against is YOU being sick or dying.

I really just wanted to share with as many people as I could, about the incredible journey I went on once my kidneys blew out in late 2006. I never set out to cure myself of arthritis, gout, headaches or anything. I only wanted to try and help my kidneys get better to avoid going on dialysis and dying. I cured myself of every disease I had. I didn't plan to become a book author either. I became one to get this information out to all of you. I'm not in it for the book sales or some more fame. My greatest thrills are hearing from those who cured themselves; knowing they have been cured!

What I did cured every disease and medical condition I had, except for high blood pressure. The damage to my kidneys caused my kidneys to stop releasing hormones that help control blood pressure. Everything is fixed and I have eliminated at least 90% of the poisons that I didn't even call poisons until the end of 2006 going into 2007. So I put all the information in this book that I needed to cure myself of all those diseases and medical conditions. And **90% of this book came from my memory of what I experienced and learned and because now I know all this stuff so well.**

There are a lot of things in this book that will improve your health and save you lots and lots of suffering, inactivity and a whole lot of money. If you really think the problem is the book, then you missed the whole point of the book. The problem is YOU. It's you that stuffed all those poisons down your throat. There is no condemnation here. It's called accepting responsibility for what you do.

You ARE responsible for stuffing that sick crap down your throat. And you can stop it. 100% guaranteed. Who's gonna stop you? Has anyone stuffed food down your throat by force? Or are you the only one stuffing anything down your throat! And when you take responsibility for what you do, then you'll get that chip on your shoulder at the grocery store against any and every product that is packed with poisons and leave them on the shelf and out of your basket. That's how you keep them out of your home and out of your body.

I don't mean to burden you with all this extra responsibility you have to take on to save your lives and avoid chronic diseases and medical conditions. I wish we had a government in this country. If we did, they would see to it that We, the People, are protected from poisons. But they only seek the approval of corporations' ability to make money. Your health is irrelevant to them. Neither the government nor the corporations will take responsibility for the obligations of their positions. And the excuse is always greed.

They're like the sickos in the music industry. If you can sell 100,000 units, just add near naked women to the cover and you can boost your sales to at least 150-175,000 units. So they add the naked women and ship it out to market. And just add high fructose corn syrup to any product and your sales go up 25%. So hey, that CAN'T be bad, because they're making money off it!

So the responsibility falls on YOU to learn how to avoid those poisons and eliminate them or at least greatly limit them. Otherwise, you honestly don't have a chance in this country. You can only get one chronic disease after another and try to find a way to cope with all the pain and suffering. **We live under the bullshit idea that we all gotta get sick to die. So we stand on that bullshit as an excuse why there's no hope of being cured and no way of avoiding disease. And it's all bullshit.**

So many of you dread the idea of the doctor telling you that you have cancer. It just doesn't have to be like that. But you can't be making excuses about putting so many poisons in your body. Even though they are FDA certified "safe" doesn't mean poisons are now safe. It means the FDA is corrupt and full of shit! They should be called the Federal Death Association, not Food and Drug Administration! You just gotta snap out of it and stop trusting the food, drinks and water to BE safe! Almost none of it is. And don't expect any of this to change. It won't. Expecting different results from the same actions is not reality. Your poison saturated food, drinks and water are FDA approved and safe.

This book is your chance to change all of that for yourself and touch the lives of so many people with help they never expected or only expected if a doctor could do it. When I look back at what I did to myself with all the "safe" poison soaked sodas and fruit juice, I am shocked at my own behavior. Not a one of you would've called it odd or wrong. Everyone actually believed I was eating very healthy. And I was! But what I was DRINKING blew my kidneys out!

I had spent a lot of time over the years making the effort to eat right. I started eating whole wheat bread in 1981. But it wasn't enough to keep me from getting a major chronic disease. And I had already accepted the headaches and heartburn as common. I never expected any of it to go away permanently.

I started my phase into chronic kidney disease with no hope for a future and the end of my life in sight just 2-3 years away and with my headaches, arthritis, gout, bleeding gums, dandruff, red itchy spots on my skin, intestinal bleeding and chronic heartburn. But I came out of it completely cured of all of it and my kidneys healed almost back to normal. If I had a book like this, I might have avoided the kidney disease altogether. Hey! If only someone would've told me WATCH WHAT YOU DRINK, I might have avoided it altogether too.

But if this had not have happened, you wouldn't be reading this book right now and you would have no hope of being cured; much less actually be cured after all the doctors told you there was no hope. I can't tell you that story. I didn't live it that way. Mine is the one where if my life was going to be saved, I HAD to do it myself. It wasn't going to happen depending on doctors. What I did worked and I am the one that is the most pleased that it did.

I would love to hear any testimonials from those who cured themselves or had their conditions improve because of what you learned from this book and put to use. Most of what I have heard comes from people outside the USA.

I want to thank my dear wife Sandra for all her support. My books are always dedicated to her. She is the perfect wife. We have never had a fight or argument in over 26 years of marriage. The things I have learned that cured me have also prevented her from getting any kind of disease. I am confident of the validity of what I have stated in this book.

I am also confident in the ability of the information to add years to the lives of those who read this book and put it to use.

So there you are! The end of this book, except for the goofy Disclaimer where I explain how I've done nothing wrong by curing myself of every chronic disease I had, then telling people in this book HOW I did that and did so without any help from doctors. I did not choose that. But it is the hand life dealt me and it is what I have already dealt with, overcome and maintained for 6 years so far.

Since publishing my first book, I've had some say I couldn't be cured since my Creatinine, by my own admission, is still usually 2.0. But since no doctor has ever seen someone do what I did, they have no standard for what a cure would be. That leaves me with no choice but to form my own opinion about that. So my opinion, which is based on facts, is that my kidney disease is cured. But the damage the enormous blood pressure did to my kidneys is not 100% repaired. Whether that can be done is yet to be seen. I'll keep working on that.

My kidneys have not gotten worse. That is for certain. My blood tests never show anything abnormal except for a persisting slight elevation in both my BUN and Creatinine levels. And the only time anything else has been out of the normal range was when I took 600mg Alpha Lipoic Acid for 3 months. Although that scared me, I lowered my Potassium from 5.6 to 4.8 in just 6 weeks when that happened. That proved my kidneys are real healthy. So no matter who ignores facts so they can pretend I am NOT cured, I no longer have chronic kidney disease or any disease.

I haven't even had a headache since the first or second month of 2007! No arthritis at all. Only an occasional slight heartburn. My EKGs show a strong healthy heart. My gums never bleed unless I poke them with a metal dental pick by accident. And no dandruff or dry skin from soaking in that chlorinated water in the shower. Damn! Even people who are considered healthy can't make those claims about dandruff, heartburn and headaches.

It does make me laugh at how hard the medical profession is still determined to keep anyone from being cured. Most of them seem threatened by the fact that people can and are being cured not only without any help from THEM, but in SPITE of them and all their efforts to keep you sick and an active customer! The struggle is theirs. And you can't let them be an obstacle to you improving your health and curing yourself. The only one that CAN stop you is YOU!

Like I practically preached to you throughout this book, YOU are the one who made YOU sick. And it is YOU that can cure yourself. And not a soul can stop you. Now see, just when you thought your life was over, you not only get to live, but get to live cured and free of disease.

So even though I was shocked and angry when the doctors threw me out of Clopton Clinic for getting better, I can't think of anything that happened to me helped more than that! Without them being total heartless frauds and mean assholes, I would most likely be dead BECAUSE of how completely worthless doctors are when you want to be cured. And to have them write on my medical records that I'm crazy for thinking THEY were going to cure me, made it crystal clear about doctors having no cures. They are OPPOSED to you being cured!

If you don't face up to these sad facts, you'll die while waiting on doctors with no cures, to cure you. I would wish you luck in curing yourself. But you don't really need luck when you learn and use proven science. Proven science works the same way 100% of the time. And that is how certain YOUR cure is as long as you at least do the major things told in this book.

And when you get the proof you are cured, open your heart and let everyone know what you have done and how they can do the same thing. As a gift to all those who buy this book or The Cure For Cancer, How to Avoid Dialysis and Cure Kidney Disease and Self-Care Heath Care Guide, I will give you a PDF version of any of these books if you email (address on title page) me with proof of purchase. You can give the PDF to anyone as long as you do not sell it.

DISCLAIMER

This book was written to guide people in doing the things that will improve their health and cure them if they are willing to do the natural things it takes to do so. While there are some facts stated in here that are critical of some things, there is absolutely no intent to defame or misrepresent the facts about these persons, companies or others. On the contrary, I intentionally left out the names of the companies saturating our food, drinks and water supplies. I did this so that no one would think that talking to these people or companies is of any real value. This book is ONLY about getting YOU cured, not fighting THEM!

So, if anyone takes anything said in this book to mean to defame, misrepresent or anything of that nature, they are only stating their opinion of what is in the book, but not stating an opinion based on facts. There are no false statements of any kind in this book. PERIOD.

But I am fully aware of how the people in the medical profession, generally and according to my own experiences, will attack and criticize anything that is not something they do and make money off of. I have no interest in their drama and choose to avoid it altogether. I have never told anyone to stop going to the doctor. On the contrary, I tell them to cure themselves WHILE they still do what the doctors say for them to do, except for the arrogant garbage about dying and there's no cure. I'm not afraid of doctors. I just know not to look to doctors or the medical profession for cures because doctors have NO cures.

No one should, in any way, take anything stated in this book as promoting or even suggesting any type of action toward any part of so-called government, companies or the likes. On the contrary, I suggest you stop buying products with the disease causing poisons pointed out in this book. And no one should be so twisted and perverted in their minds to claim that Individuals do not have the Right to protect ourselves from disease causing poisons and all poisons.

This book places absolutely ZERO HOPE that food companies will ever make the choices to remove the deadly, addicting, disease causing poisons from their products. So the only choice we have is to freely share the knowledge individuals need to avoid the poisons in food and drink products. Just because doctors and the rest of the medical profession don't get to make money off the diseases I cure or prevent and never have, doesn't constitute any illegal or inappropriate act or acts; regardless of how their unbridled greed causes them to tell more lies to try and protect all their current lies they tell the Public.

There are only a rare few places in this book where any text was copied from a web site and pasted into this book. These few places were from Public sites with no copyright stated. This was only done for accuracy of rules and policies. Anyone who thinks their copyright has been violated in any way, can contact me for a quick and amicable solution in your favor.

Knowledge is Power. And that absolute Power scares those who know they are poisoning us to death and those who prolong our diseases to maximize their incomes. So inventing false claims against me and this book are what they do to try and preserve their jobs and keep all of us suffering and dying to insure their bloated incomes. It is up to each of you to choose to value your own lives and health over preserving their jobs, incomes, lies and unbridled greed.

We just want to keep living. And as long as you do what this book says, that is going to happen for you. I only advise you to avoid these poison happy greedy corporations. You can hope some doctors will start curing people some day. But that is not reality at the time. But at least you have a way to cure yourself. And that is what this book is for and what I want for all of you.

There can be no legitimate claim against me for wanting people cured and doing something about it. On the contrary, join me in praising cures. Cures saved my life and empowered me to overcome sickness and Death. This is what America use to be all about. True Americans succeed because we have to. Failure is not an option.

I am living proof of that. So be well and live long.

Best regards,
Author and Publisher Terry Cooksey

The Facebook page for this book is:
www.facebook.com/Natural.Healing.BOOK.of.CURES

Alphabetical Index

CPSIA information can be obtained at www.ICGtesting.com
Printed in the USA
BVOW01s0057131214

379270BV00005B/15/P

9 781939 147400